ADh-3886

A pt
8/08

D0466291

DISCARD

613.7   Phillips, Shawn.
PHI
           Strength for life.

DATE			

SANTA CRUZ PUBLIC LIBRARY
SANTA CRUZ, CALIFORNIA

BAKER & TAYLOR

ALSO BY SHAWN PHILLIPS

*ABSolution: The Practical Solution for
Building Your Best Abs*

Strength for Life

Shawn Phillips

Strength for Life

The Fitness Plan for the Best of Your Life

BALLANTINE BOOKS | NEW YORK

No book can replace the diagnostic expertise and medical advice of a trusted physician. Please be certain to consult with your doctor before making any decisions that affect your health, particularly if you suffer from any medical condition or have any symptom that may require treatment.

Copyright © 2008 by Shawn Phillips

All rights reserved.

Published in the United States by Ballantine Books,
an imprint of The Random House Publishing Group,
a division of Random House, Inc., New York.

BALLANTINE and colophon are registered trademarks of Random House, Inc.

LIBRARY OF CONGRESS CATALOGING-IN-PUBLICATION DATA
Phillips, Shawn.
    Strength for life : the fitness plan for the best of your life / Shawn Phillips.
        p. cm.
    Includes index.
    ISBN 978-0-345-49846-5
    1. Physical fitness.   2. Exercise.   3. Muscle strength.   4. Health.
I. Title.
    RA781.P55 2008
    613.7—dc22   2007042064

Printed in the United States of America on acid-free paper

www.ballantinebooks.com

9 8 7 6 5 4 3 2 1

First Edition

To my children, Nathaniel and Lilly,
and our newest generation;
may you live with strength.

Preface

Cautious not to make extended eye contact, I scanned the overflowing room full of familiar faces spanning back to my earliest childhood memories. The room seemed to spin. I paused to catch my breath, steadied my feet firmly on the ground, and forged on. Feeling as if in a dream, I stepped behind the podium, gripped the microphone, and began to speak.

As I delivered my father's eulogy the room was silent one moment, erupting in laughter the next. Laughter might have seemed inappropriate to some, but this is precisely how my dad, "B. P." Phillips, would have wanted it: The lighter moments brought much-needed relief from the intense pain. I held nothing back. If ever there was a time for strength, this was it.

That May afternoon, I stood atop a mountain overlooking my hometown of Golden, Colorado. It was the culmination of a whirlwind stretch in which I turned forty, welcomed into the world my first child, Nathaniel, and married my love, Angie. Now I was saying good-bye to my father at the too-young age of 62.

As a family we'd enjoyed a decade-long run atop the health and fitness world. My brother at the helm, we rode EAS to the summit, creating books, magazines—even a movie that changed the face of fitness forever. Naively, I imagined that success meant immunity to this sort of tragedy. "It can't happen to us," I believed.

I was wrong.

I could not change the fact that my dad was gone. What I could choose was my perception of it; whether it "happened to me," the victim's view, or if it simply happened. By fully accepting the loss, albeit with a great deal of pain, I found the strength to create a new future. The opportunity was there, as it is in every moment in life, to choose strength and to move forward.

Courage is not the absence of fear, it's strength in the presence of it. It's stepping into the fire and embracing all life has to offer. It's in moments like these, when life kicks you square in the teeth and you bounce back, that you begin to suspect the depth of your true potential.

The moments when life challenges you to step forward, to take control, can be turning points—as turning points are simply an opportunity to change, accepted. Most people wait for change to be thrust upon them. Rather than choosing to take action, being resolute and resourceful, they live in reaction, waiting until it's a matter of life or death.

These people go their entire lives playing it safe, waiting for the right moment to show up strong and realize their potential. They fear they lack the necessary strength, whether of character, determination, heart, body, or mind, to seize the opportunity—even when it's right there in front of them. "What if it's the wrong path?" they ask. They say to themselves, "Perhaps the time isn't right . . . I'll get to it later."

Can you recall a time when you let an opportunity slip by, when you could have taken decisive action but didn't? We all know that experience. Now recall a time when you flexed your muscles of willpower and desire, moving forward with uncommon resolve. Can you just feel the strength, the clarity, the power that you manifested with focused intention? That power is always available to you. Sadly, we don't use it more often.

It's easy to pretend there's plenty of time. I know, I was sure I'd have more time with my father. Procrastination is dangerous. Whatever you've dreamed of doing, being, or seeing, now is the time to be the creator of your life. Make this moment count, act as if it is all you have.

The way I see it, there are but two kinds of people—those who've done remarkable things to change the world, and those who've yet to awaken their capacity for strength and let their greatness shine. When you choose strength, strength chooses you.

After many years of helping people live their best lives, I've come to accept that you cannot build a strong body with a weak mind, nor can you build a strong "you" with a weak heart or spirit. It begins on the inside and radiates into every aspect of your life. The book you hold in your hands has the capacity to help you chisel your abs, build your biceps, sculpt your glutes, balance your mind, open your heart, and reach deep inside to the foundation of that universal source of power I call *strength*.

Shawn Phillips
Golden, Colorado

Contents

Introduction

If the idea of having a lean, strong, beautifully fit body; of feeling great with more energy and even looking years younger grabs your interest—great news: You've just taken the first step toward your absolute best life.

Strength for Life contains easy-to-follow proven principles and practices that can empower you to transform your life. Whether you just need to drop a few pounds, sculpt and shape, boost your confidence, lift your energy, or create a brand-new you, I invite you to take the decisive next step with me and dare to discover just how truly amazing looking and feeling great can be.

Perhaps you're thinking, "Sure, I'd enjoy swapping some weight for shape and I'm in for more energy and self-confidence, but I've got to know: What's it going to take? I'm very busy—there is so little free time. Will this be something I can do? It best be fast and easy or I'll drop off."

At one time or another we've all felt the draw of the quick fix. The hope is that the picture-perfect body might come in a pill, that you can diet your way thin without exercise, or even that cardio alone can shape your body strong. If you're still being held back by any of these fitness fantasies, the book you hold in your hands will set you free.

What if forging your body stronger and leaner was something you truly enjoyed doing? There would be no reason to celebrate your remarkable discipline, for you'd look forward to it the way avid golfers do a tee time.

What if I were to show you how to get motivated and stay motivated for a lifetime of strength and fitness?

What if I were to show you how you could fall in love with not just the feeling of being fit but the art of training itself—so that you could have the body, the energy, and all that comes with it—without relying on boatloads of discipline?

Would you step up for that?

What if at the same time you train your body strong, you are also strengthening your capacity to focus and concentrate, becoming more centered, boosting your confidence and performance in work, relationships, and life? Imagine how amazing it could feel to know that your entire life, not just your belt line, is enhanced by your fitness practice.

What if you were to discover a depth and center to strength training that you've only associated with yoga and martial arts?

What if I were to show you a surefire way to end dieting, forever. And give you a simple practice that can change your entire relationship with food?

Would that inspire you to commit?

What if you could swap ten pounds of unwanted body fat for three pounds of lean, strong, energy-burning muscle in about 30 minutes per day? What if your new, stronger, leaner body burned more calories driving your car or just sitting each day than it did previously running three to five miles a day?

What if you were to discover that strength training is not just for men or athletes but is the real secret for women to sculpt a shape they previously only dreamed of?

And what if you enjoyed the time economy of stacking the benefits of strengthening your mind while training your body—for double the results? In this time-crunched world, there's tremendous value to one activity producing multiple benefits.

Sound good?

The breakthrough program I've put forth in *Strength for Life* is going to help you sculpt your body lean and do much more. It's a guide to life at full strength. I'll show you how to start strong, get strong, and stay strong by igniting your inner fire of motivation, helping you to channel it, to transform it, and finally to live a transformed life.

THE TRANSFORMATION OF FITNESS

There was a time not long ago when *transformation* was how butterflies came to be—not how people came out of their shells—when getting fit most commonly involved some wearisome mix of dieting and jogging. The idea that you could radically reshape and revitalize your body without counting calories, without dieting, and with only a brief amount of cardio and strength training, was unheard of. The logic flew in the face of widely accepted reality, which a yet-to-be-well-known fitness expert and author was about to transform.

Armed with volumes of real-world proof in hundreds of visually stunning *before* and *after* photos of lives changed, the transformation began in the spring of 1999. By year's end this fitness book dominated the bookstore aisles where diet books had previously reigned and had risen to #1 on the *New York Times* bestseller list.

A perennial bestseller since, having sold many millions of copies, *Body-for-LIFE* is the most successful and arguably the most significant fitness book ever. Millions have been inspired to transform their bodies and lives through this landmark 12-week exercise and nutrition program.

The creator: none other than my brother, Bill Phillips. I'm proud of Bill's success and privileged to have been a part of a better than decade-long run of success leading a fitness revolution, redefining the way people approach training, nutrition, and life. Along with millions of readers, I owe my brother an enormous debt of gratitude for the pioneering book, the original transformation program, and the mission set forth that he continues today.

If you've experienced *Body-for-LIFE,* you can expect to discover a sense of the familiar in this program. But make no mistake: *Strength for Life* is a work of my passion, knowledge, and life experience. Unlike the many *Body-for-LIFE* imitators, this book is more than a lateral move, another sideways step. Rather than simply another take on the 12-week process of transforming your body, *Body-for-LIFE*'s strong suit, this program elevates and continues to guide those who've transformed while bringing an entirely new dimension to the process.

TRANSFORMATION VS. CHANGE

As we near the tenth anniversary of *Body-for-LIFE,* there's no debating the fact that it has positively impacted millions of lives. Yet, for all that it's done, not every person has enjoyed a successful transformation. And even among those who've enjoyed remarkable transformations, it's a small percentage of individuals who have sustained the fitness levels captured in their "after photos."

I've had the pleasure of speaking with hundreds of people and reading thousands of stories of men and women who've followed a 12-week Transformation program. Nearly every one of them fit into one of three distinct groups: the *Frustrated,* the *Enthusiasts,* and the *Transformed.*

The Frustrated

A common story I hear from people who failed to complete a Transformation is they began week one with great enthusiasm but found themselves drifting away before completion. They speak of struggling with motivation, being too busy, and simply not having the necessary energy.

I call this group the Frustrated, because they carry the burden of believing that they're part of a small minority who didn't achieve the success seen in the "before and after" photos. What these readers don't know is that they had great company and their failure to finish a Transformation is likely not an issue of desire or motivation.

Like the majority of Americans, the Frustrated are often sleep-deprived and eating poorly, which means they are undernourished and overstressed. When they add the physical demands of a Transformation program that would invigorate a "ready" body, their bodies break down rather than become stronger.

Stress and fatigue will silently sabotage even the strongest motivation. As a result, people start skipping workouts and then stop altogether. Sadly, many of these people are left believing they have failed when it's not their fault at all. Depleted when they began, their bodies incapable of responding to the demands, their wisest path forward would have been a step back— to recover first.

Unfortunately, this deprived, fatigued state is more the rule than the exception. That's why it's crucial for *everyone* to invest a couple short weeks in preparation before embarking on a Transformation.

The Enthusiasts

One of the greatest strengths of *Body-for-LIFE* is that it inspires rabid enthusiasm. However, elevated by their new body and level of fitness, many people come to the end of the 12-week Transformation and, absent any other course of action, promptly start all over again. And without the necessary down time for full recovery, the very thing that triggers your body to get leaner and stronger can quickly start working against you. As a result, your body begins to break down muscle, dissolving all of your hard-earned achievements.

What Enthusiasts are not aware of is that a Transformation is an intensive period of conditioning designed specifically to transform and is not intended as a sustainable lifestyle. Both physically and mentally demanding, the potential for burnout and overtraining increases with each week one pushes beyond the initial twelve. And doing another Transformation after completing one is like riding the Tour de France back-to-back, a feat even the world's top cyclists would not attempt.

A simple course of action can help Enthusiasts maintain the progress they enjoyed in their Transformation and keep their momentum going strong. More on this in a moment.

The Transformed

The most fascinating group of the three are those who didn't just change their body and snap a photo. In the process of Transformation something clicked inside—they truly Transformed.

It's important to note here that there is a difference between *change* and *Transformation*. Where change is change, I define *Transformation* as "significant and lasting change." It's change that doesn't snap back to the way it was before. Take, for example, learning to read—that's transformative. You don't go back to the way you were before, being unable to read.

A Transformed person has become a strong positive force, continually striving to improve. They are on a quest for growth, and it's no longer an effort—for being their best has become the way they *do* life.

The unique experience of each of these groups has provided valuable lessons and inspired the total Transformation solution that is *Strength for Life:* Start Strong, Get Strong, and Stay Strong.

THE THREE PHASES TO FULL STRENGTH

To maximize your Transformation and support your continuing success, the *Strength for Life* program provides an elegant, sound, three-phase approach. First there's the vital, yet overlooked, 12-day *Start Strong* preparation phase that I call *Base Camp.* This primes your body and mind for the most successful transformation possible. It's also a time you can use to fully prepare and refine your vision and inspiration for your transformation.

With Base Camp complete, your body rejuvenated, your motivation on high, your goals clearly in view, you charge into *Get Strong,* the full-strength version of the classic 12-week Transformation program.

Concise, efficient, and effective, this 12-week *Transformation Training Camp* integrates the clarity and wisdom of the original with a modern-day approach that suits the increasing demands of life at any age—especially the challenges faced by the working adult, parent, and professional.

Now that you've discovered the freedom and energy of a renewed life in a rejuvenated body, the next step is to live it. What is it that happens for the Transformed group? How do the switches get flipped in such a way as to create their life anew? In Week 13 and Beyond you and I will cocreate a sustainable plan, a lifestyle that supports the new you and a lifetime of *sustainable* energy and strength. This is the 12-month *Stay Strong* phase.

A DECADE OF CHANGE

After a decade of Transformations, much has been learned about training, nutrition, and fitness. Yet the fundamentals of *Body-for-LIFE* have stood rock-solid, becoming more widely accepted and endorsed by science. *Strength for Life* embraces the accumulated wisdom while elevating the experience to the next level. It's a stand-alone system. You need not have mastered *Body-for-LIFE* or any fitness program to experience success with *Strength for Life*.

From my vantage point, looking back nearly a decade, I smile thinking about my early experimentation with the training program that became the *Body-for-LIFE* workout. My office door led to an elaborate, fully equipped gym where, after long days, I relished spending an hour or so training at peak intensity. It was my meditation and my rejuvenation all at once. At that time my training was such that I honestly feared *Body-for-LIFE* to be overly simplistic. Today, I find myself saluting its simplicity, while embracing even greater simplicity.

Now in my forties, I have a wife, Angie, and my two children, Nathaniel and Lilly, and a new company, Phillips Performance Nutrition. Gone are the days of training and working whenever I chose, for as long as I desired. My life, both more rewarding and more complex than ever, has given me an entirely new understanding of the challenges of staying fit amid the many demands of family and work life that I only thought I understood years ago.

I've continued to evolve my nutrition and training to best serve my fitness goals within the context of my life goals. To me, strength is not superficially determined by what I see in the mirror or how many hundreds of pounds I can lift. It's about feeling great, staying young, and enjoying energy to burn.

That brings me to the central promises of *Strength for Life,* which are *efficiency* and *effectiveness.* From the perspective of an entrepreneur, a father, and a husband—with access to a decade of transformational wisdom and the culmination of my more than twenty years in strength and fitness—this program is designed to provide you with the absolute maximum results in the absolute minimum of time.

At the heart of the *Strength for Life* program is the revolutionary training system I created that integrates the wisdom and insight embodied in yoga, meditation, and the martial arts with the numerous physical benefits of strength training. Called Focus Intensity Training™ (FIT for short), it is the synthesis of ancient wisdom with modern science into a graceful, powerful, body–mind practice.

The result is an entirely new training experience that is at once more effective, refreshing, and engaging. And while for many people its selling point will be the superior effectiveness and results, the real surprise inside may well be its impact not just on the body, but on your inner state—emotionally uplifting, strengthening your awareness and presence, as well as bolstering your overall well-being. Add to that, as your mental focus develops, you will find yourself training in an enjoyable "flow" state.

Yes, that's right. In the final analysis it's all about enjoying the process—having whatever you do regularly bring pleasure. Even training. If there's one thing I've learned in helping people live stronger lives, it's that we simply don't stick with anything, regardless of how "good for us" it is, if we do not enjoy it.

If in the past you've struggled with strength training, even knowing its importance, FIT can inspire and set you free. It provides a spark, a depth that is a true breakthrough in training. FIT is like electricity and you are the lightbulb—it will turn you on and have you radiating.

MY PROMISE TO YOU FOR YOUR BEST LIFE

The *Strength for Life* program along with the knowledge, wisdom, and guidance contained in the pages that follow can and will transform your life. But there is a catch. The catch is you. That's right: You are the wild card, the variable I can't control. Regardless of what I say, in the final assessment, your success is in your hands.

Bruce Lee said it well in these words: "Knowing is not enough, you must apply; willing is not enough, you must do." You can count on me to reach in and help fire you up, to keep you moving and inspired for greatness, but ultimately it's up to you.

This opportunity for change is your invitation to create a Turning Point. Only you can accept it and take the first step toward making the possibility a reality. Take a moment, look deep into your heart, and choose to step into your strength. I'm confident you're ready for *Strength for Life*—and I'm ready to be your guide.

How strong are you? Let's find out.

A Time for Strength

If we are strong,
our strength will speak for itself.
If we are weak,
words will be of no help.
—JOHN FITZGERALD KENNEDY

CHAPTER 1

Beyond Health

HOW HEALTHY ARE YOU?

Just for a moment, let's forget about being lean, strong, and fit and just talk health.

Do you value your health?

If your answer is a resounding *"Yes!"* you're not alone. America is on a health kick, and I believe it's killing us.

That's right. I believe our obsession with health is a dangerous, debilitating, disastrous mind-set that may be undermining the very fabric of our nation—as well as your own health. I'm confident, in a few moments, you'll agree.

In fact, we're losing a battle that is costing us our health, wealth, and ultimately our strength as a country. The obesity epidemic is spiraling out of control. We're working harder and longer, eating more, and moving less. Kids now stare at screens rather than engage in real-life activities, at least until their parents commandeer the television for their own use.

The numbers are startling. According to the National Center for Health Statistics, about 30 percent of U.S. adults 20 and older are obese and 65 percent are either overweight or obese. One out of five ages 12 to 19 is now considered obese.

Simply being overweight, let alone obese, increases the likelihood of developing numerous health conditions, including diabetes, high blood pressure, heart disease, stroke, breathing problems such as asthma and sleep apnea, some cancers, and osteoarthritis, among others. Yet, the greatest impact is simply on quality of life.

Studies suggest that more than 400,000 people die each year from causes related to poor diet and physical inactivity. That's 17 percent of all deaths. Only tobacco use, according to research by the National Institutes of Health, accounts for more fatalities.

Though the death toll from most preventable causes decreased in the decade between 1990 and 2000, obesity and inactivity deaths went up by 33 percent. By 2010, poor diet and physical inactivity likely will overtake smoking as the leading cause of preventable death.

Recently we crossed a tipping point where, for the first time in recorded history, the youngest generation of children is now expected to live shorter lives than their parents, even though medical technology continues to advance and we know far more about the impact of poor diet and inactivity than ever before.

The ranks of the uninsured grow each year, as does the staggering costs of health coverage for employers. Health care costs have been rising faster than the rest of the U.S. economy for many years, as they continue to consume a larger share of family budgets.

Unless something changes, our already precarious health care system will collapse and millions will face financial ruin and premature death. No one is immune to the impact.

If you're in a group health care program at work, the rates are determined by factoring everyone in your office—including the obese and the smokers. It's not like auto or life insurance, where you catch a break for safe driving or clean living. You're penalized for the sins of your associates.

As of 2007, obesity was costing the United States $130 billion in direct medical costs each year. It's not a stretch to suggest that the figure soon could soar to $1 trillion annually. Businesses, already straining to provide employees health coverage, will be forced to drop coverage or go outside our borders, a choice more companies have already made. Many doctors are leaving the profession, because insurance companies increasingly are covering less of their services. What's most unsettling is that the greatest impact will most likely happen to us in ways we can't even begin to imagine.

Most of us know something is not quite right, and many can quote a stat or two about the crisis, but it's little more than cocktail conversation. It's not quite personal, even when we *are* part of the problem. Studies have shown that 64 percent of obese people don't think they are obese—"it's the other guy or gal. Not me."

Like the parable of the frog that stayed in the pot of water until it was boiling, it's getting hotter and hotter but we don't seem to mind. It hasn't yet occurred to us that it might be time to jump.

Why worry, so long as you've got your health, right?

THE PARADOX OF HEALTH

What is health, really? Think about how you might explain health to a three-year-old. Perhaps you would reach for some buzzwords like "fit," "well," or "sound." Eventually you'll come to the clarity that we all do and just say it like it is, health is the "opposite of sick."

For most all of us health is subconsciously, if not consciously, defined as the "absence of disease." Technically, this is an accurate definition. Heck, even the esteemed *Merriam-Webster's* dictionary defines health as "freedom from disease."

For most people, health is less a goal than it is a nice idea, a concept. Saving 10 percent of your income, losing 10 pounds—those are goals. Instead we talk about health, eat a few veggies, slip in and out of a diet, and try to avoid the doctor. We may "get serious"—this lasts a few weeks, perhaps months. Alas, there's work, the kids, so much to do—we get drawn back into life. No harm, though, you're healthy and will get around to it later.

So few truly value this elusive thing called health.

Given the way most people view health, barring any sudden, tragic diagnosis, you're "healthy." You could be 80 pounds over your "desirable" weight, snacking on Ding-Dongs while lounging at home watching television, and self-assessment would be: Cancer? Not me. Tumors or broken bones? Negative. All systems check in as free from disease: "Healthy!"

As in this example, the remarkable goal-seeking radar we humans have is letting you down because you seem to be working perfectly. You see, it's masterfully designed to move you *to* your goal, not beyond it. Once your subconscious checks off a goal (in this case "free from disease") as attained, your drive slips into neutral and nothing more happens. The status quo settles in.

We've been so oversaturated by "healthy" media messages that we've stopped thinking critically about the actual meaning of health. It's become something we check off our "to do list" more than a state of being. This lack of clarity has us walking a tightrope between "healthy" and "not healthy." As long as people *feel* healthy, they take little action to be more than that. Their goal realized, they're in a comfort zone, oblivious to the dangers of their sedentary, reactive lifestyle.

The tragic reality is that most people never make real or lasting change until it's absolutely necessary—until they're ill or faced with a serious health scare, and even then they don't always change. Cigarette smokers are sometimes unwilling to kick the habit even after a lung cancer diagnosis. Remarkably, some smokers assume they're healthy until told otherwise. Why not? All systems were reporting back "healthy."

Here's the real message you should be receiving when it comes to your health: "Houston, we have a problem."

You see, for most people health is less the presence of something great than the absence of being ill. It's settling for "good enough."

This is why our fascination with health is dangerous. How can it be that millions of people in this country think about, worry about, and appraise their health—and yet we find ourselves in a spiral of decline facing an enormous crisis of health? Isn't our obsession with health supposed to reverse these trends?

Certainly there are good intentions to report on and some pockets of people who are getting stronger and healthier, but for the most part nothing is changing—at least not for the better.

I care about your health and the well-being of our country and world, but the harsh reality is that *health is not enough*. I want more for you, for your family, and I know you can have it. It's all here for your taking. That is precisely why I'm asking you to join me on this journey *beyond health*—beyond the "good enough" survival mentality—to a life of abundant energy, vitality, and strength.

STRENGTH IS PRESENCE

Where health is no more than the *absence* of disease, strength is the *presence* of abundant energy—a capacity to be a force in your world. It includes health and at the same time so much more; it's being healthy and flowing with energy, power, and confidence.

To live with strength is to choose abundance—it's more than avoiding illness or simply getting by, it's a higher state of energy and life for those who have set their sights beyond health. Call it "optimal health" or "strength," its hallmark is a desire to improve; there is no settling for the status quo.

Without strength, there's never enough energy to go around or enough hours in your day. You can't get it all done. People in this position consider the process of strengthening their bodies a luxury. There's just not enough time.

Strength is that something extra; the mental, physical, emotional reserve—the fuel that makes for an extraordinary life. Where "health" is like living paycheck to paycheck, strength is money in the bank—a reserve. Strength is true wealth.

Together, we stand at a turning point in our existence, a time when we must find the strength to change: to change the way we think, the way we eat, the way we relate to our bodies, the entire way we embrace our planet and world. As formidable as these changes are, all change begins with the strength and the courage to master your own life challenges.

You may choose to live your life at full strength for yourself in order to do more, be more,

---

HEALTH VS. STRENGTH

HEALTH ⠂⠂⠂⠂➤ STRENGTH

MONEY ⠂⠂⠂⠂➤ WEALTH

EFFECT ⠂⠂⠂⠂➤ CAUSE

SCARCITY ⠂⠂⠂⠂➤ ABUNDANCE

---

and have more of everything. You may do it for your family, who will benefit greatly from the care and maintenance of the vehicle you call you. Or you may choose to do it for your country, which ultimately bears the burden of the weak and frail.

Your body, the only one you will ever have, is the foundation for your life. And it's either an anchor limiting your freedom and potential, or a source of radiant energy, vitality, and joy, elevating your life and the lives of those around you. It's your choice. Will your body be a source of strength, from which you will impact the world, or an obstacle, preventing you from your dreams and desires?

As my friend, NFL Hall of Fame quarterback John Elway, is fond of saying, "If you're going to set a goal, aim high!"

My advice to you is to aim high; aim for strength.

CHAPTER 2

The Shape of Your Life

Whether you're tall, short, thin, curvy, or stout—whatever shape you see in the mirror—the shape of your life will likely look much the same as every other life. It rises up, arcs over and through your peak, and descends.

If you were to graph the strength, energy and vitality of your life, it would look like the cross section of a speed bump. You're born weak and helpless, spend the first two decades of life growing stronger, enjoying vibrant energy. There's a leveling off as you reach a comfortable cruising altitude. Then the inevitable: In spite of your attempts to defy it, the descent begins. You spend the rest of your life walking the "tightrope of health," quietly hoping and praying that you don't slip back to weak and helpless.

Where are you along this normal curve of life? Here's a simple way to gauge it. Think back to your last birthday. Was it an exciting celebration, or has it become a dreaded annual event, similar to tax day?

If you've "celebrated" a fortieth birthday like I have, you know it can be a startling experience. It's not so much the stigma attached to 40, or the good-natured grief you receive on your birthday, but the realization that your physical prime is no longer in your future. In an instant you've gone from seeing your best on the horizon, to watching it shrink in the rearview mirror.

At this point your body has been quietly stockpiling fat and divesting lean muscle, strength, and energy for more than a decade. The redistribution of fat, especially in the common problem areas—the midsection and thighs—is increasingly apparent. If you've ignored your nutrition and exercise up until this point, the neglect is visible for all to see.

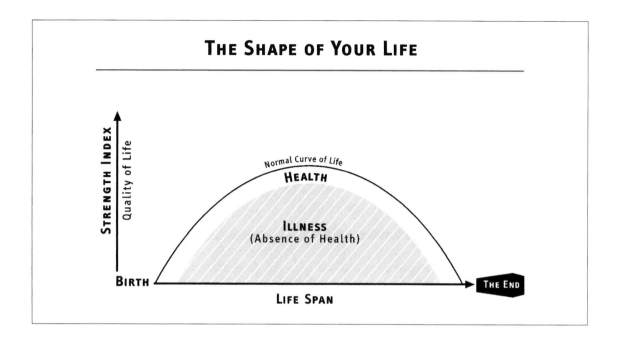

THE SHAPE OF YOUR LIFE

STRENGTH INDEX / Quality of Life

Normal Curve of Life

HEALTH

ILLNESS
(Absence of Health)

BIRTH

THE END

LIFE SPAN

Yet somehow in the midst of these disturbing life changes, most manage to ignore them. This is easy to do if you've yet to reach your fourth decade milestone—for even thirty-nine and a half is "thirty-something." You're still young and healthy. No reason for you to worry yet, right?

The day this rationalization fails, and you are no longer able to ignore your declining physical condition, is a difficult day indeed. For the unprepared, midlife can bring trepidation and discomfort. Some seek temporary relief in the likes of a new Corvette, Botox, or cosmetic surgery. Yet, try as you may, you will eventually reach the point where you simply can't buff it out any longer.

Now, let me make something clear: This is not a book about being forty-something, but rather a book by a forty-something from the pinnacle of life, who's going strong and has another forty (at least) strong years ahead. With more than two decades' experience in strength and fitness, I see both the ascent and the descent on the curve of life with stunning clarity. From this perspective, I'm confident I can help you shape your best life, whether you're 25, 75, or anywhere in between.

THE DESCENT BEGINS

Physical decline actually begins long before you see its many signs. Starting in your midtwenties you're losing about a pound of lean, life-enhancing muscle per year. This loss of muscle usually goes unnoticed for many years, as the weight is replaced with more than a pound of fat, which takes up five times more space on your body. Hence, the reason you can weigh the same and still find your clothes won't fit. As a result, your shape gradually morphs, softens, and widens as your energy, strength, and vitality fade.

By the time the average, modestly active person debates going to their twentieth high school reunion, they can expect to have packed on 20 or 30 pounds of fat, even though the scale is showing a not-so-bad 10 to 15 pounds (remember you're losing muscle). If you're not eating well, these startling numbers could be a best-case scenario.

You guessed it; things do get worse. In the absence of a significant change in lifestyle the decline continues to gain speed. By your midfifties you can expect the above numbers to double. This could mean a staggering 60 pounds of fat gained and over 30 pounds of muscle lost for a man and an equally disturbing 35 and 15 for a woman. As difficult as this should be for you to grasp, if you're not there yet, consider that in the case of a woman, it represents less than one pound of fat gained per year since high school graduation.

Any way you slice it, this sort of physical morphing is a major blow to your quality of life: It's damaging to your health, metabolism, self-image, career, and even to your relationships. It could mean heart disease, diabetes, or worse. Every aspect of your life is impacted. And as if that's not unsettling enough, this places you dead center in the target market for an enormously profitable sector of the pharmaceutical industry. That's right, companies are banking on your illness and decline.

Eventually, there comes a point in every life where you can no longer ignore the enormous and expanding gap between the life you could be living and the life you've settled for.

This gap I'm describing, between your current state and a life of strength, is not strictly a function of age; even many 18 year-olds could be living a better, fuller, stronger life. Ideally, your prime window for adding lean muscle is between the ages of 18 and 30. Having said that, every day of your life that you're not actively engaged in staying fit, eating well, and strengthening your body the gap grows.

You may feel too busy to give fitness your full attention. Then one morning as you're getting dressed you catch a glimpse of what looked to be Marge Simpson's, or worse yet, Homer's, naked body in the mirror. It'll be years before you walk past that mirror naked again.

Whether you face reality head-on and make a life change or deny your responsibility, you've made a choice. The way I see it you choose either a life of abundant strength and energy or you're living in the gap, far beneath the quality of life you could be enjoying.

The choice you've made up to this point is clear. Should you desire any further support for choosing the high road, consider the following checklist of common symptoms you might be needlessly tolerating:

COMMON SYMPTOMS EXPERIENCED IN THE GAP

- Gradual weight gain, especially in your problem areas
- Noticeable drop in energy levels after lunch and in late afternoons
- Frequent cravings for snacks, sweets, or other junk food
- A disappointing and declining sex life
- A reliance on coffee to get you going and more to keep you going
- Tired earlier in the evenings yet often unable to sleep
- The feeling that you've aged 3 years in the last 17 months

Are any of these symptoms familiar? If so, you're not alone. Millions of Americans have come to accept this steep decline, and the needless suffering it causes, as the normal curve of life—the "price of aging." We give it no more thought or resistance than we do the setting of the sun each evening.

Barely into our thirties, at the first sign of a body ache or the arrival of a couple extra pounds, the inner dialogue begins, "You're not getting any younger." Aging, like gravity, is a given. We don't see it, so we don't question it. We just know that when dropped, a rock hits the ground, and we too willingly accept the same fate.

Not only does this decline of your physical capacity have a negative impact on career, family, and your quality of life, there's an even greater price we all pay for this needless loss. Just when people have the most to offer the world, when they've moved beyond the "me plan" and are inspired to make their mark, this decline in energy and vitality can rob them of their ability to make meaningful contributions to family, friends, and communities.

We all lose something invaluable when we lose our strength.

But I've got some good news for you: If you've been tolerating any of these symptoms, you can stop now.

This normal curve of life I've just described, and which most of us have long ago accepted as a given, is not accurate. It's a myth, a story our beliefs have given life.

In reality, these symptoms—and the declining body that goes with them—are much more likely the result of physical, mental, and emotional fatigue from being overworked, overstressed, overtired, overfed, and undernourished, and just plain out of shape. All things you can change now, at any age.

This news may not be easy to accept, for it does appear that this decline of life is "the way things are." Just as it was once a given that a boat made of steel could not float and that man would never fly, change involves challenging the assumptions we've mistaken for reality; and this is one of them.

Consider for a moment just how deeply ingrained and powerful our beliefs are around this so-called normal curve of life. It's so ingrained in our culture and minds that when anyone, anywhere along the path, breaks from the norm, we recognize them as exceptional. It could be the 15-year-old art prodigy, the 44-year-old major league baseball pitcher, the 52-year-old cyclist who bikes across America faster than twenty-somethings, or a 90-year-old barefoot water-skier who lives with the energy and zeal of a teenager.

Sure, at first glance these do seem extraordinary—but what is it that makes them so? You got it: what you believe to be ordinary. Just for a moment, try on the idea that these examples are not something so exceptional but more the expression of your full potential—the path we could all choose.

Yes, you might say, but these people are special, gifted. Well, consider this: What if you're gifted too? How would you know for sure? Have you exhausted the possibility that with all your focus, intensity, and heart, you are as gifted as they are?

You're Never Too Old To Gain Strength

The Noll Laboratory for Human Performance compared young men with men between ages 45 and 60 and found that percentage of body fat, along with aerobic capacity, was not related to age but rather the amount of time spent training the body. The Human Nutrition Research Center on Aging found muscle growth in people ranging from 60 to 96 years old was statistically equivalent to younger people doing the same amount of training with their bodies.

One of the fastest rising and most debilitating conditions of aging is sarcopenia, a disease in which a person loses large amounts of muscle and strength. As this research indicates, the symptoms of aging are less dependent on age and more related to lifestyle. Thus, a lifestyle that includes regularly engaging one's body with strength training can make you strong now and keep you going strong for life.

Most people are settling for less than their potential, for less strength, energy, and vitality than they can have and deserve. To accept life anywhere below our fullest potential is to be living in the gap, blindly accepting "what is" without ever deeply considering "what could be."

It doesn't have to be this way. You can create a second coming, a new, leaner, stronger more confident you, rejuvenating your body, mind, and spirit with the sound, simple intelligent plan that is *Strength for Life*.

SPANNING THE GAP: THE S CURVE OF LIFE

I call this resurgence the "S curve" of Life. Instead of accepting the normal curve, the arcing speed bump paradigm, gradually going downhill, this is your opportunity to step up and choose the higher path—to stop living in the gap being less than you can be. The evidence is strong and science validates what millions of Transformation success stories have revealed: "typical signs of aging" are more the result of how you live than how long you've lived.

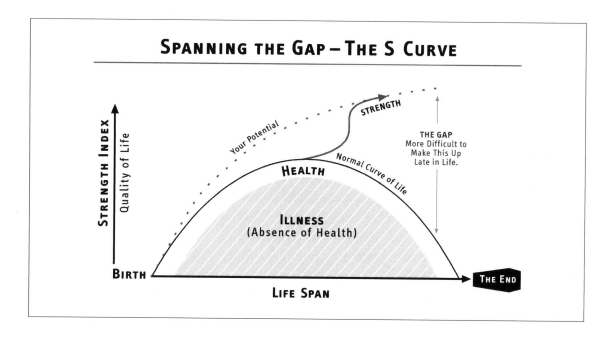

No matter where you are in life, whether twenty-two, forty-two, or sixty-two and beyond, you have the power to decide how you're going to live today—and for the rest of your life. From this day forward, with the *Strength for Life* program, you can choose a higher trajectory for your life and start growing younger, stronger, and leaner today and each day forward.

Choose a life at full strength. An extraordinary life with a future more brilliant than your past awaits you.

CHAPTER 3

A Strong Mind for a Strong Body

Can you focus? I mean really focus. Are you able to free yourself from the distraction of noise and constant chatter bouncing around in your head for even a few minutes?

Go ahead. Give it a try. I'll wait. For just two minutes sit quietly, clear your mind of all activity—be free from any thought as you focus on your breathing. The clock is ticking. Now close your eyes.

Welcome back. How'd it go?

Were you startled by the amount of noise in your mind? If it sounded like you were receiving three television stations, a traffic report, along with the last song you heard before getting out of the car, you're not alone. That's the way our minds are most of the time, only we don't notice because we're constantly distracted by the very same relentless stream of stimuli. For most of us it's tough to focus on anything, let alone something as subtle as your own breathing.

If you struggled with this brief experience with focus, that's okay. Please don't let it be discouraging. While it may seem like a simple thing to do, the power of focus takes training and repetition to develop, as any seasoned meditator can attest.

While the idea of spending hours on a cushion may not sound particularly inviting, you can still enjoy the many rewards of a clear, calm, focused mind—a mind free from the stress-creating, energy-draining mental chatter that is the norm. In a moment, I'll share with you a revolutionary method that can help you develop laserlike mental focus—strengthening your mind as you strengthen your body.

Focus is the concentration of attention to the exclusion of all else. It means putting everything you have into what you're doing at this very second—whether it's on work, training, nutrition, a friend or loved one. When you're focused, you're not thinking about the past or future. Nothing else enters your mind.

We live in a world that demands our attention, compromises our focus, and steals precious time. Our minds must withstand a constant assault of stimuli. Focus frees you from stress, cultivates energy, and offers you a sanctuary of sanity—a place to renew and connect with your innerstrength. Focus is a master skill of an extraordinary life.

Perhaps more than any other factor, it is the mastery of your focus, which precedes the mastery of your energy—that separates the average performers from the peak performers in life. The freedom to place your focused attention where you want it, when you want it, offers a competitive advantage in a world where the average attention span is measured in seconds, not minutes. It's precisely this skill that has so many high-profile leaders adopting meditation practices. Steve Jobs of Apple, music icons Rick Rubin and Russell Simmons, Oprah, Bill Ford of Ford Motor Co., and the Clintons are a few of the prominent names that belong to the rapidly growing population of Americans—currently reported to be more than 20 million—who have embraced the practice of meditation.

Typically, the mention of meditation conjures up images of a kind, elderly gentleman sitting on a cushion. In truth meditation is anything that brings you to the present moment and keeps you there. It's what best-selling author and teacher Eckhart Tolle is instructing us to do when he so eloquently says, "Focus your attention on the Now." With anticipation of our future and memories of the past streaming through our minds like a dozen movies, the last place we're likely to find ourselves is in the Now, regardless of how quiet the room is.

Whether you've embraced it or not, when *Time* magazine in 2003 featured a woman meditating on the cover along with an article on the science of meditation, it became increasingly difficult to ignore its growing impact. And the mounting body of science continues to support the finding that the more we practice meditation—the more we focus on the Now—the stronger we are physically, emotionally, and mentally.

A recent study at Massachusetts General Hospital found that meditating actually increases the density of neural connections in the brain, which lends yet another piece of evidence to the growing body of research uncovering the many benefits of meditation. Hundreds of studies conducted at over 200 independent universities in over 30 countries around the world have established our first modern understanding of the neurological, physiological, and psychological impacts of meditation. Here are just a few of the many benefits of focusing on the Now:

- **Increases the growth of new brain cells**
- **Increases your IQ and Emotional Intelligence scores**

- **Increases broad comprehension and productivity**
- **Improves mental focus, memory recall, and decision making**
- **Decreases stress, anxiety, and depression**
- **Reduces free radicals, heart rate, and biological aging***
- **Improves quality of and ability to sleep**

* **Meditators in their midfifties were found to be biologically twelve years younger than their nonmeditating peers.**

THE FEELING OF FOCUS

We've all been there, in total focus. Most people associate intense concentration, or being focused, with times of great productivity. This view tends to overlook the deepest, most blissful states of focus you may ever know, the times of your life that have little to do with getting anything done but everything to do with being present in the moment.

These moments could be as simple as being lost in a breathtaking sunset over the ocean, or life-transforming events like the birth of your child, your wedding, a first kiss, or any life achievement that puts you on top of the world.

Think about a high point that first comes up for you. Get a clear picture in your mind. Recall the vivid detail. How does the air smell? Is there a cool breeze or warm sun on your skin? What sounds are present?

When you're there, recall what was on your mind. Were you jumping out of a perfectly good airplane (with a chute on your back, of course) and thinking about making the car payment, an upcoming meeting, or when you could catch your favorite TV show?

What else were you thinking of? The answer: nothing. You weren't thinking what the next day would bring or what happened last week. You weren't even thinking about the present moment; you simply were the moment. Any thought would have taken you away from being in the Now.

The prominent philosopher and author, Ken Wilber, speaks to these moments of total focus most eloquently in his book, *No Boundary*: "Lost in a sunset; transfixed by the play of moonlight on a crystal dark pond which possesses no bottom; floated out of self and time in the enraptured embrace of a loved one; caught and held still bound by the crack of thunder echoing through mists of rain. Who has not touched the timeless?"

Real focus is effortless, when—if only for an instant—we stop "doing life" and step fully into being alive. For most people these moments are reserved for special events. For some, they require a high-risk adventure to experience; for others a new relationship is needed to feel it again. However it occurs, this amazing force arrives when you break free from the chains of the busy mind—when you're so focused in the Now that the walls that usually protect and deflect are down.

THE STRENGTH OF FOCUS

If there's one thing I've done differently in my training over the past twenty years compared to almost everyone I know, it's to apply a high degree of focus and intensity to each repetition of every set of every exercise. Applying specific techniques that isolate my muscles and concentrate the power of my mind and body has allowed me to enjoy extraordinary results from ordinary exercises.

As I discovered some years ago, in the practice of strengthening my body, training had become my own preferred form of meditation. The specific techniques I've used over the years are captured in the unique discipline of strength training I call Focus Intensity Training (FIT). Applying these transformative techniques, as you will learn to in this program, allows you to make an extraordinary leap in the results and effectiveness of your workouts.

Here's a quick illustration of how dramatically FIT can change things. Take your right arm and extend it out, with your palm open. Now close your palm, as if you're gripping a dumbbell. It may help to grab something nearby with that hand first, such as a pen or cell phone. Now curl the arm as if you're performing a biceps curl.

No big deal, right? In fact, that exercise probably seemed rather useless. Unfortunately, this is the same approach most people take in the gym.

Now let's do it again. This time, however, as you begin to curl your arm, contract (squeeze) your biceps and touch your left index finger to the center of your right biceps. Then picture a red hot marble just under this point of contact and focus your eyes on this same spot. As you contract your biceps slowly, continue to deepen your complete concentration on this single spot of your muscle. When you reach the peak, the fully contracted position, hold it. For about ten seconds continue to increase your focus and intensity. Then release.

Did you feel the difference? I'll bet you did.

You might find that your biceps feels hot—not just inside but to the touch. If nothing else, you no doubt feel your biceps more intensely than you did during the first attempt since you stepped up your focus and intensity with a few simple techniques you'll learn more about in Chapter 11.

Having guided thousands of people through this eye-opening exercise, I'm familiar with the look of amazement and the "ah-ha" sound that goes along with what you've just experienced. The change in the way your biceps feels can be big—when all you've done is elevate your typical unfocused, drifting state of mind and apply focus and intensity to this very basic movement.

An evolution in strength training, FIT benefits from and embraces the fact that your mind and body are not two separate entities but rather function as one interconnected, interdependent system. And the benefits of skillfully engaging them in harmony are extraordinary.

While modern medicine is just beginning to consider the possibility of a connection between mind and body, in the ancient traditions from the East, their unity has never been a question. The integration of mind and body in the quest for optimal health (a.k.a. strength) is not a novel concept. The Greeks too have long advocated the balance between mind and body as the ultimate aim of man. This philosophy is captured in the well-known phrase, *"Mens sana in corpore sano,"* which translates to "A healthy mind in a healthy body." With the demands of life in the twenty-first century, I contend nothing less than "A strong mind in a strong body" will do.

By skillfully engaging them in harmony, you will realize not twice the benefits, but many times more. Fully engaging your mind during your training strengthens your ability to be focused in the moment. Engaging the full energy of your body with a focused mind strengthens the wiring that powers the mind–muscle link. This is a best-of-both-worlds approach: FIT blends active meditation with strength training—strengthening your power to focus while strengthening your body.

This stacking of benefits for body and mind in training has been going on for centuries in other physical disciplines including yoga and the martial arts. For example, tai chi is a moving meditation that requires the practitioner to focus on the whole body flowing seamlessly as a unified force. Similarly, many forms of dance integrate the movement of the body with a highly focused mind.

While there are a number of physical practices that harmonize body–mind, FIT integrates this ancient wisdom with the relatively modern practice of strength training. In comparison to some forms of martial arts and yoga that date back several thousand years, weight lifting as practiced today is barely more than one hundred years young.

In the following table you'll see how this integrated form of strength training that embodies meditation compares to other disciplines, both modern and ancient. Upon review I'm sure you'll agree that while there's merit to all of these approaches, FIT provides several distinct advantages.

A Comparison of Physical Practices on Body & Mind

	Weight Lifting	Yoga	Meditation	Running	FIT®
Strength & Muscle	★★★★	★★	-	★	★★★★
Focus & Concentration	★	★★★★	★★★★	★★	★★★★
Energy	★★★	★★★★	★★	★★★	★★★★
Endurance	★	★★	★	★★★★	★★
Flexibility	★★	★★★★	-	★	★★★
Body/Mind Integration	★	★★★★	★★★★	★★	★★★★

In FIT, you find techniques such as breathing, concentration of attention, deep relaxation and surrender, flow of energy, grounding, and others that are found in the great Eastern practices. The common element is the full engagement of body and mind as one.

Unfortunately, a large number of those who do exercise with weights regularly do so with only moderate effectiveness. Rather than fully engaging themselves in the activity, they go at it halfheartedly or simply space out.

Take a look around your gym. More often than not you'll see people more focused on counting reps and watching others than on their own training. This casual, going-through-the-motions approach may be the single greatest obstacle to a strong body and a strong mind.

FIT is at the heart of the training you will do. Its aim is to develop not simply your physical strength but integral strength: strength of body, mind, emotions, and more. Think of this new style as strength training from the inside out—integral strength training.

By focusing the combined energy of the mind and body, it's as if you're going from the light of an ordinary fluorescent bulb to the concentrated intensity of a laser beam. And for many there's no better place to develop this ability to focus than during intense physical training.

As you begin to master FIT, harnessing your power to focus, expect to enjoy an increasing state of flow during your training. This is that "in the zone" state that athletes often speak of—the place where time seems to stop and what once was work becomes effortless grace. As you progress through this program, there will come a point where the *doing* training transforms into *being*—where you are one with the moment and every subtle nuance of it. This is the unmistakable moment of freedom.

FIT Research

In a pilot study of FIT conducted by my wife, Angie, as part of her master's thesis in somatic (body) psychology, fourteen men and women practiced FIT regularly for 30 days. In just that short period of time, they discovered increased strength and energy and a feeling of greater intensity during workouts. They also found they had clearer minds, higher levels of motivation, greater enjoyment while training, higher levels of self-confidence, as well as an increase in focus and concentration into their daily lives that transcended the gym.

Consider what you might experience as you embrace and conquer the *Strength for Life* program.

Think of a time when you've been "in the zone," so deeply involved in an activity that time seemed to stop. You were flowing with energy and confidence, free of doubt and fear. That's focus. Now imagine how powerful it would be if you were in this deep state of focus throughout every workout. Consider how powerful it would be to bring this intensity of focus to every part of your life. You'd be more productive, getting more done in less time with less effort; more present in relationships, more attentive, more caring. You may even enjoy every moment of life a little more.

How will the power of focus change your life?

CHAPTER 4

The Undeniable Case for Strength

You can hardly go a single day without being reminded that as a nation we're getting fatter—and we're all suffering for it. You read some of it right here in Chapter 1. It's a very real issue that is deservedly getting much attention.

The obesity epidemic is receiving a lot of airtime. You hear the wisdom every day, with weight loss and health gurus urging people to "get off the couch, set the chips and soda down, and *start exercising!*"

Still, Americans continue to pack on the pounds, and I believe I may have uncovered the cause. So I have a slightly different message to offer: *Stop exercising!*

Yes, you read that right; I'm absolutely convinced that exercise is failing us—or more accurately, exercise *has* failed to produce the anticipated positive impact on the ever-increasing number of overweight Americans.

We've got more people exercising than ever—running, doing yoga, belonging to gyms, attending aerobics classes, buying in-home exercise equipment, and engaging in new forms of cardio exercise. And yet we're getting more and more unhealthy.

Go into one of the modern fitness center metropolises and take a look around. My guess is, what you'll see is a pretty standard scene—loads of cardio machines, lots of people moving, reading, talking, socializing, watching TVs, or watching others. In another area, some barbells and dumbbells, a load of big machines (a few that look intimidating), and a few people staring blankly, some talking and others engaged in moderate circuit programs on the machines.

These people are simply going through the motions, dutifully performing exercises with the type of enthusiasm they bring to household chores. This dull, uninspired shuffle called "exercise," this failure to train with a sufficient level of focus and intensity, is the greatest obstacle to developing the results most profess to be seeking.

Though often used interchangeably by others, *exercising* and *training* are distinctly different. Exercise is movement without purpose, motion without direction. It's what my grandmother does when she walks around the block.

Now, I am for anything that elevates the heart rate and gets a body moving, and this is all that some people are capable of. Exercise is a grueling activity that requires great discipline, an obligation: "I should be doing this." In contrast, training is powered by an inspired vision: "I feel strong, fit, and alive!"

I'm sure you've seen people training in those same gyms too. You'll recognize them as the few who truly look like they mean business. Head down, focused, intense, driven with purpose. They're not unfriendly people, just "in the zone."

For a clear example of the difference between exercising and training, consider the fact that athletes don't go to "exercise camp," they go to training camp. Why? Because they are "in training"; focused on achieving specific results, which fuels an intense drive and motivation.

In this program I'll show you how to bring that same intensity and purpose to your cardio training as well your strength training. Training is a mind-set, the way in which you approach any exercise you do, be it a set of bench presses or a session on a treadmill. Understanding this distinction will be as transformative to your results as the training itself.

I believe in and am a proponent of cardiovascular training; I do it and have come to enjoy it. However, you'll note the *Strength for Life* program emphasizes strength training.

If you could have only one reason to make strength training part of your fitness life, you might try this fact: It is the *only* way to reshape your body. Attempting to transform a body with cardio alone is futile. As my brother Bill is fond of saying, if you're shaped like a pear and do nothing but cardio training, you might lose some weight. But you'll just end up looking like a smaller pear.

Strength for Life is not an exercise regimen but a

TRAINING VS. EXERCISE

TRAINING
- Motivated by a "Want"
- With Goals and Purpose
- Focus, Intense, Engaging
- Meaures Feedback
- Produces State of "Flow"

EXERCISE
- Done for Own Sake
- Without Goals, Purpose
- In Response to "Need"
- Lacks Intensity
- Can Be Boring

training program. If you are serious about transforming your body and life, if you have any desire to make measurable change, if you want your time in the gym to be efficient and effective, stop wasting your time exercising and start training!

THE STRENGTH OF TRAINING

I still remember being fifteen years old when I saw the movie *Pumping Iron*. In it, future Terminator and California governor Arnold Schwarzenegger passionately compared the feeling of intense weight training to one of life's greatest pleasures. Convincing? Let's just say Arnold had this teenager considering a new path. There's no question that Arnold's rise through Hollywood and into politics can in part be credited to the charisma, confidence, and inner strength that he's forged through years of dedicated strength training.

Long considered essential for bodybuilders and athletes, lifting weights has been increasingly scientifically recognized for its positive impact on physical and mental well-being and is viewed now as critical to lifelong vitality and overall quality of life at any age.

Yet, weight lifting remains an enigma: an activity without the structure of organized sports and lacking the mystique of yoga or the history of martial arts. There are a lot of myths and misunderstandings about weight training.

When I'm teaching seminars on Focus Intensity Training, the first thing I do is create an opening for the audience to embrace a new possibility for weight lifting—or *strength* training, as I prefer to call it. For most, it never occurs to them that strength training might offer lifelong benefits.

Up in front of the room, a set of dumbbells at my side, I begin by asking, "What comes to your mind when you see these?"

It doesn't take long before the emotional descriptions start flying. I capture them as fast as I can write on a whiteboard.

"Build muscle?" huffs a thirty-something woman. "That's exactly what I *don't* want. I need to lose weight, not add it!"

A midforties yoga instructor nods. "Weight lifting? No thanks!" she says. "Why would I want to look like a hulking man?"

A thin, frail man pipes up next. "I don't have the time to go to the gym. I'm in great shape from running three miles a day."

"You couldn't pay me to go to one of those gyms full of self-centered people," hollers a woman from the back row.

"I just started a new exercise program guaranteed to give me six-pack abs!" boasts a loyal reader of a popular fitness magazine.

The responses are almost always the same, including these popular descriptions of weight training: shallow, narcissistic, boring, for men or athletes only. When they're done venting, I shrug my shoulders and admit, "You're absolutely right. Strength training *can be* all of these things. It also can be unnerving, intimidating, and downright uncomfortable."

There's an audible sigh of relief from the audience.

"You've made some great points," I continue. "Of course, these same feelings arise for some when confronted with a black diamond ski slope, the first tee box of a golf course, or a yoga class."

I'll concede the desire for a strong, lean, fit body can be *perceived* as shallow as driving a Mercedes, as vain as the mat-packing yoga devotee, or as macho as an intense black belt. But even if it were true, none of this prevents strength training from becoming a deeply engaging, transformative practice for you.

I never cease to be amazed at the passionate responses I get from this one simple question. I'd expect to hear such heated viewpoints if I brought up a polarizing political issue, but for a couple of dumbbells? How can people get so worked up about something as simple as strength training?

Perhaps it's in part that people don't generally like to exercise. They see it as a burden. They understand conceptually that exercise is good for them and may even like the idea of dropping a few pounds. But they're uncomfortable with the notion of *building* muscle, as they are more focused on *losing* weight—thus they cling to myths of dieting, cardio, and weight loss pills.

No one has ever made it clear to them that adding lean muscle can be the fastest and easiest route to achieve what most people want: a sculpted, lean, fat-burning physique that's full of energy, vitality, and strength to make you look and feel great.

However, this isn't just about boosting the ego. Strength has a profound impact on your emotional state. Sure, it feels good to look good, but it's more about the positive energy that's created. When you feel strong, you walk taller and make better eye contact. You command a room and have greater clarity in all areas of your life.

In the world of neuroscience, Hebb's Law suggests that brain states (feelings) that occur together repeatedly tend to become grafted together. That means when you feel confident and powerful during a moment of strong physical expression—i.e., strength training—it is reinforced with each rep and set. These feelings of confidence, power, and strength will become a present and accessible part of your daily life experience, and not just in the gym. Strength training, especially Focus Intensity Training, will hardwire this feeling of confidence until it becomes part of the very fiber of your being.

Donny Deutsch, the marketing guru turned talk show host, a man who discovered the joy of strength in his forties, beautifully describes the feeling of "being strong" in his book *Often Wrong, Never in Doubt*:

> It's visceral . . . There is incredible power in the ability to sit at a table and know "I'm strong." That image of yourself extends to all areas of your professional and personal life. Physical well-being says you are disciplined, you are a winner.

Muscle gives your body a shape. It conveys an aura of strength and confidence, even when you're dressed in winter clothing. With strength, you carry yourself with a purpose, you look and feel like the force you truly are.

There was a time in my youth when how I looked was the primary driver of my training, but today I go a little deeper. Strength training helps me be more effective and confident. It influences the way I feel every day, and can do the same for you.

THE 7 WONDERS OF STRENGTH

1. Muscle Is the Engine of Youth

Muscle is the engine of youth, and strength training is the most effective way to build muscle. As current research is uncovering, biological aging and the loss of functional strength have less to do with your chronological age than they do with time spent training and engaging the body for physical growth and development.

Strength training is the most effective way of slowing down and even reversing the process of aging. In their book *Biomarkers,* William J. Evans and Irwin H. Rosenburg covered 10 "biomarkers," key physiological measures of the aging process. All 10, the authors said, could be favorably altered through strength training alone.

The 10 biomarkers are: muscle mass, strength, basal metabolic rate, body fat percentage, aerobic capacity, blood sugar tolerance, cholesterol, blood pressure, bone density, and the ability to regulate body temperature. The authors believe, as I do, that muscle mass and strength are the two most significant variables determining the quality of your life.

This does not mean you're going to train with the goal of developing big, showy muscles, the sort of muscles people tend to visualize when they hear "muscle mass." Rather, I'd like you to look at muscle as *lean* body weight that keeps you active, fit, and energized, as opposed to the flab people believe is inevitable as they age.

2. Strength Training Builds a Strong Foundation

Numerous studies show that adults who exercise have greater bone mineral density (BMD) than less active people. Weight-bearing activities such as strength training produce greater BMD than nonimpact or low-intensity activities such as swimming or yoga.

I'm a fan of swimming and yoga. But strength training is *the* best way to build strong bones, tendons, ligaments, and muscle, which are all essential to your physical foundation. Unless you strength-train, you'll start to lose bone density after your teenage years and become susceptible to osteoporosis, which is not exclusive to the elderly or to women.

Strength training also protects against injury by increasing the flexibility of joints. Studies suggest that Olympic weight lifters are second only to gymnasts when it comes to flexibility because so many lifts enhance flexibility as they build strength. Unquestionably, the idea that strength training makes people stiff and rigid has been dispelled as a complete myth.

3. Strength Training Is Good for Your Mind and Mood

Thomas Jefferson once remarked that "a strong body makes the mind strong." If you've studied the life of the third U.S. president, you know he was a true Renaissance man and fitness enthusiast who lived to be eighty-three, well beyond the life span of folks born in the middle of the eighteenth century. You'd be hard pressed to name an American who has made as many significant contributions to so many fields, including the guiding principles that still govern the United States today. Clearly T.J. was on to something when he drew a connection between physical and mental strength.

Strength training stimulates endorphins, neurotransmitters, and neurotrophic growth factors your brain thrives on, making you feel good during and immediately following training. Scientists are now discovering long-term positive effects of regular strength training: It makes your neurons more robust while improving blood flow, oxygen, and nutrients to your brain.

Michael Craig Miller, M.D., editor in chief of the *Harvard Mental Health Letter,* summarizes what scientists have been uncovering for several decades: Regular training "improves your mood, decreases anxiety, improves sleep and resilience in the face of stress and raises self-esteem." He adds that exercise itself makes for a "pretty good antidepressant too, equal to drugs or psychotherapy in some studies."

When your body is strong, firing on all cylinders, you can't help but feel more focused and, yes, smarter. Focus Intensity Training will further enhance these effects. You will increase your ability to concentrate and improve your emotional and psychological well-being.

It all comes down to this: When you feel more confident and capable of doing anything, you're going to be happier. Strength training is a powerfully effective way to get there.

4. Muscles Shape You Smaller

Many people, not exclusively women, resist strength training because they're concerned it's going to make them "look big" or muscle-bound.

Here's the irony: Strength training actually shapes you smaller. That's because a pound of muscle is much smaller and takes up less space than a pound of fat. A pound of fat is about the size of a cantaloupe. In contrast, a pound of lean muscle is about the size of a baseball. Using this analogy, imagine how amazing you would look and feel if you swap 20 pounds of fat (think 20 cantaloupes) for five pounds of lean shape-defining muscle (think 5 baseballs).

Not only that, these five lean pounds will be evenly dispersed around your body, not residing, as fat does, in a few problem areas. Five pounds is just enough to give you some shape. It's not the sort of volume to add size.

5. Muscle Makes the Scale Irrelevant

When people focus solely on cardio training, losing weight, and counting calories, they often become obsessed with scale weight. A five-pound gain or loss is cause for rejoicing or despair. For some the scale can become like a daily mood ring. The scale looks only at weight—it does not take into consideration the composition of that weight: whether it's water, fat, or precious lean muscle.

A loss of muscle reduces the metabolism and accelerates fat gain even more. That's why dieting without strength training will never result in permanent weight loss. Not only have you not created additional lean muscle to burn calories, you've likely reduced a portion of that valuable resource. This is why most dieters who have lost some fat will gain it back faster.

Because a pound of fat takes up much more space than a pound of muscle (as described above), you must begin to see body weight in terms of body composition. A 150-pound woman who has only 25 pounds of fat will fit easily into a dress that a 135-pound woman with 50 pounds of fat cannot. Use a mirror or be in tune with the way your clothes fit—and be kind. When you have a lean, strong body, the number on the scale is irrelevant.

6. Muscle Is Money in the Bank

The goal of any long-term financial plan is to create assets that generate income with little to no effort on your part. This security, for many people, offers the freedom to enjoy your retirement or to do whatever you like, whenever you like.

Having muscle is the same type of asset for your body. It's like having money in the bank. For every pound of muscle you gain, you're able to burn 35 to 50 calories more per day—

with no added effort. That's because lean muscle boosts metabolism, which in turn can burn fat. One pound of muscle consumes the caloric equivalent of five pounds of fat in just one year.

Adding just one pound of muscle will enable you to burn on average an additional 18,250 calories per year. A pound of body fat burns just 700 calories over the course of a year. This is why fat begets more fat. It doesn't take many calories to fuel body fat, and what's not used is stored as, you guessed it, more fat!

Let's say you've added 10 pounds of lean muscle to your body. Just carrying those 10 pounds around for daily activities, not including exercise or training, can burn on average an additional 500 calories each day. That's over 180,000 extra calories in a year, the amount of calories stored in about 52 pounds of fat! It's also the equivalent (estimated, of course) of running four miles each day for a year.

Does it take effort to add that lean muscle? Of course it does, much like the accumulation of financial assets takes time and effort. But by making a modest investment, as you'll do in this program, you'll be rewarded handsomely.

7. Muscle Enhances and Prolongs Life

The list of life-enhancing benefits of having added lean muscle is staggering. Muscle regulates and stabilizes blood sugar levels, which not only enhances fat reduction but can prevent the onset of diabetes. Muscle also contributes to lower cholesterol levels and helps prevent cardio-vascular disease.

Muscle does not only make you look good, it takes an active role in supporting your well-being. Success begets success, for those who have lean muscle tend to get leaner and stronger. The more muscle you have, the faster and hotter your metabolism burns, and the easier it will be for you to swap fat for lean muscle.

If you add five pounds of lean muscle, you'll find yourself able to eat more freely and still regulate or even lose fat. You'll have a wider margin of error. Your muscle will actively help regulate the glucose in your system and thus limit fat accumulation and promote fat loss.

When people lose muscle, either through inactivity, chronic dieting, or excessive cardiovascular training, they may eventually end up suffering from a debilitating disease called sarcopenia; an incapacitating loss of muscle. An increasingly common and devastating condition in the elderly, sarcopenia is typically associated with aging. Today, sedentary lifestyles are resulting in an increase of middle-age victims. It bears noting that this disease is not a normal part of aging but results from a lifestyle of inactivity.

When you have lean muscle, you've made a long-term investment in your quality and longevity of life.

Jan: A Solid Case Study

Now let's go back to my friends in the seminar so I can give you a real-life example of how adding just a few pounds of muscle can completely transform your body.

Jan is a 38-year-old wife and mother of two who works full time. She would like to lose 20 pounds and has been bouncing up and down 10 pounds with various diets for years. She does yoga once or twice a week and has been "wogging" (walk/jogging) for 30 minutes every day at lunch. She says she doesn't have the time to belong to a gym. Besides, she doesn't want to build muscle. She wants to "lose inches and get toned."

In listening to Jan, I'm moved by her motivation and commitment. She's putting forth considerable effort in her quest for fitness. I assure her that based on what I know so far, I can help her achieve her goal *and* save her a tremendous amount of time and effort.

I explain that her program of "wogging" for 30 or even 60 minutes daily is helpful for her health, at least under our maintain-the-status-quo definition of health, but not enough to make lasting change.

"Don't worry, though," I say, sensing her anxiety. "It's not more time and effort you need. It's more effective, targeted training."

Next, I break it to her that there's actually no such thing as "toned muscle." The idea that you can work a muscle at moderate intensity for a long time for tone is a myth. Tone is the product of strong, conditioned muscle, best achieved through intense strength training and reduced body fat.

As for the benefit of yoga, there are some challenging styles of yoga that strengthen, but for the most part yoga is practiced for flexibility as well as opening the body and mind.

The path Jan has chosen to take in her fitness efforts is a common one. It's the result of people doing the best with the information they have. It seems like a sensible solution. The problem is, it's plagued by a high rate of failure because people quickly stop making progress. They lose motivation and quit. Thus, the weight returns and people like Jan throw up their hands in frustration.

At least Jan has the sense to exercise. Dieting alone is ever more challenging, especially when you consider that 90 percent of dieters eventually gain all or more of the weight back. Add to this the fact that more than 50 percent of the weight lost while dieting is from lean muscle. That makes it harder to lose weight and keep it off, due to the fact that there's less muscle to keep it off!

That's worth repeating. The dieter may lose weight, but at the same time a smaller amount of food can make them gain weight, because their metabolism is slowing. It's a self-limiting, frustrating, and challenging path.

I assure Jan that I can show her a sound, sensible way in which she can achieve her 20-pound

continued on next page

weight loss, and do so in about the same amount of time each day that she's committing to now. By following the *Strength for Life* plan, she can lose her 20 pounds within a few months and be nearly 100 percent certain that it is 20 pounds of fat that she has lost, not just temporary fluid loss, and definitely not a loss of lean muscle.

Now that I've got her interest and attention, I tell her, with great enthusiasm, that the *only* sure way to drop 20 pounds and maintain her new body is with an effective strength training program. She looks at me with a combination of indignation and disbelief. I get the sense she's feeling duped.

I assure her that I'm on her side, that it does work and will work for her. Still, Jan is reluctant to abandon her belief in cardio as the key to being thin. She says she can feel it working, that sweating is the same as burning fat, and that she's afraid of lifting weights.

I ask her, "Are you willing to trade 20 pounds of fat for 4 pounds of lean muscle?"

I explain that Focus Intensity Training will provide many of the rewards of yoga while also sculpting her body. The 4 pounds of muscle she needs is merely enough to help her achieve the shape and "toned" look she is after, while it serves to help her lose and keep off the 20 pounds of fat.

"While you're engaged in your daily activities, that 4 pounds of new muscle is burning calories at the rate of 200 a day. That's about the amount you burn if you run two miles as fast as you possibly can. So carrying those four pounds of muscle is the equivalent of running two miles a day, every day."

Jan had mentioned that she has a friend who exercises five days a week on a treadmill. "You can tell her, 'I run my two miles seven days a week. I run at top speed, and I never have to leave my desk to do it!' "

It's that simple. A mere four pounds of muscle can have a significant impact on our lives.

I can hear the reactions in the seminar room now. "Four extra pounds of muscle would make me look like a hulk!"

I understand the momentary disbelief, but let's look at this logically. As you already know, muscle is much more dense than fat, so a pound of muscle is much smaller than a pound of fat. Furthermore, you're trading 20 pounds of fat for your 4 pounds of much smaller muscle. Think about what it might look like if you were to take four pounds of thinly sliced turkey (lean, of course!) and wrap yourself with a thin layer. Spread it around your arms, biceps, triceps, chest, shoulders, and legs. You'd run out of turkey long before you covered your major muscles with even one thin slice. In other words, 4 pounds of muscle will increase your size by less than one-sixteenth of an inch, while trimming inches of fat, mostly from the problem areas.

There is yet another benefit from building your four pounds of muscle. Not only does this muscle burn the caloric equivalent of a two-mile run every day, but the calories required to build the muscle in the first place are far more than you can imagine and will result in drawing down fat reserves.

It's common for people who have not committed to strength training consistently to oversimplify the act of building lean muscle. They assume it's as easy as adding fat, but it's really quite a feat of biological engineering. While a pound of muscle contains 3,500 calories of energy, the number of calories required to assemble that pound of muscle is many times greater.

The formation of a pound of muscle is analogous to building the Great Pyramids of Egypt. The pyramids were not carved out of rock that was already there, but assembled by men lifting countless rocks into place. So it is with building a muscle.

If you look at the big picture—the energy required to build muscle, the training needed, the effort exerted, the elevated metabolism—and all the while your food intake remains static, you can expect to lose up to a pound—perhaps two—of fat per week. That might not seem as dramatic as some infomercials or miracle weight-loss drugs, but this isn't random weight loss. It's real *fat* loss, and there's a good chance that when you're doing all the right things, it will be permanent fat loss.

As I finish this brief explanation, Jan heads for the exit. Unsure if I've upset her, I ask, "Where are you heading?"

"To the gym," she says.

Base Camp:
12 Days That Will Recharge
Your Body and Mind

You gain strength, courage, and confidence
by every experience in which you
really stop to look fear in the face and
do the thing you think you cannot do.
—ELEANOR ROOSEVELT

CHAPTER 5

Rest, Renew, Reboot

When was the last time you woke up fully rested—eager and energized to start your day? Think back; perhaps it was day six of a seven-day vacation when you were last in balance, enjoying your natural flow of energy.

As rare as this surplus of energy is for most, think of how a child awakens each day. My young son, Nathaniel, pops out of bed every morning with his tank full. No need for a grande coffee or anything to get him going. He's ready and eager to greet the thrilling day ahead.

What was the first sound you heard this morning when you awoke? Was it a radio station blasting or the screeching sound of an alarm buzzer tossing your cells into their own alarm state? For most of us, living the American Dream, it's a moderate-voltage wake-up followed by our favorite brew, a shower, and whatever it takes to get us back on the warrior path.

We've become so accustomed to living in a fatigued, compromised energy state brought on by chronic stress that we fail to consider that it could be any other way. It's become the norm. And many actually embrace it, using it to get them moving. This chronic stress drains us from the inside, stealing our energy and vitality. Combine this with poor nutrition and lack of sleep, as it often is, you've got a recipe for physical, mental, and emotional depletion—a virtual house of cards ready to collapse at any moment.

Then one day, elevated by a sense of urgency, you decide from your overstressed, overcommitted state that now is the time to get in shape. You take on a fitness plan hoping to correct this physical wreck in mid-collision.

"Sure, you can do it all," you tell yourself. The big red S on your chest carefully concealed, you dive into a Transformation—like you'd dive into a swimming pool—although in your current state it's as if you're diving in with both hands tied behind your back and cement galoshes on. To your great astonishment, you sink like a rock, thanks to your compromised state and lack of preparation.

Enter into your upcoming Transformation physically, mentally, and emotionally exhausted, and your results will reflect your depleted state. You'll likely wind up another casualty of the mysterious "loss of motivation or discipline."

It's common even among those who most eagerly dive into a Transformation to hit an invisible wall. It may arise as low motivation, which is the fatigue taking over. It's like an inner intelligence saying, "enough already." For adding more stress, even a "positive stress" like a Transformation, only further compromises an already overloaded system.

If you're one of the many who have lived the story of having "failed to Transform," here's some good news: What you actually failed to do was prepare. It's not that you failed to close strong, but failed to start strong.

The reality is that the intensity and demands of a Transformation are often too great for those who enter unprepared. The credit for uncovering this weak link in Transformation programs goes to my friend and colleague Tom Bilella, D.C., M.S., a prominent whole-life specialist who operates the Nutrition Treatment Center in Red Bank, New Jersey.

It was in his clinic that he revealed the problem he referred to as the "depletion syndrome"—an invisible hurdle that was impeding people's progress mid-Transformation.

Following the release of *Body-for-LIFE,* Tom's clinic was flooded with clients taking on the challenge, eager to be one of the next success stories. About half of his clients were enjoying the sort of progress one would expect, while the other half experienced quite the opposite. Rather than getting stronger and leaner, they were exhausted, drained, and frustrated. They were doing the very same Transformation—all the right things—yet this group was neither losing weight nor gaining muscle.

Tom recounts one of the stories:

> The fatigue on her face and in her voice was apparent. I concluded she
> needed to recover her energy and get back to baseline. She was deter-
> mined to complete her 12 weeks of Transformation. Convinced that she
> had to back off—in an instant I stopped treating her as a fitness client
> and began treating her like any other case of chronic stress. I used tests
> to show her what was taking place on a cellular level. Then I explained
> that she was in a severe state of stress that was affecting her body's abil-

ity to recover—what's called a "catabolic state." And to continue training and excessively limiting nutrition would only stress her body further.

With this strong persuasion, Tom convinced his client to take two weeks off to rest and recharge. To help her revitalize and get her body running smoothly, he provided a simple set of guidelines much like those I will share with you in a moment.

Two weeks later, Tom's client came back for her appointment. Tom recalled, "I barely recognized her. She was exuberant, positive . . . shining with energy . . . like a different person. With two weeks of minimal activity, she'd added nearly two pounds of lean muscle and produced a measurable drop in body fat percentage. In every way she was coming back to life."

Rebound Strong with Super-Compensation

Let's say you are a muscle. A good-looking muscle with a great smile and terrific personality, but a muscle nonetheless. Oh yes, and you're also a muscle belonging to a strong, healthy person who trains you.

First, you undergo intense stress as you are trained. On a cellular level this causes you—the muscle—to break down, leaving you weak and compromised. Following training, you anxiously await the much needed flood of vital nutrients that, along with the necessary rest, will trigger your repair and full recovery.

Soon after you begin receiving that nutrition and rest, your strength begins to return as you rebuild. This continues until you've reached your previous baseline—the condition you were in prior to your last training session. And then something extraordinary happens: The strength keeps building beyond your previous best—building a larger reservoir of strength should you once again face a similar stress.

Now you're at the peak of recovery, on top of the world, fed, rested, and stronger than before. This process of rebuilding yourself stronger, shifting to a higher capacity, is called *Super-Compensation*.

Your body, while certainly more complex on a macro scale, can recover from a depleted, stressed state in much the same way as a muscle. As the effects of chronic stress are addressed, as they are here with the Five Reboot Rules, your body will start coming back to baseline, back to balance and a full, vibrant life. When it does, you may regain muscle that's been lost under stress and feel your metabolism start to crank back up.

As it is for the trained muscle, a period of rest, recovery, and renewal is essential for your body—and is especially true prior to a Transformation. Where muscle typically requires 36 to 48 hours to recover following training, your body requires more time. The 12 days of Base Camp is the perfect boost to get your body heading in the right direction.

Add muscle and lose fat without exercising—sounds too good to be true, right?

Actually, it makes perfect sense when you understand the inner workings of the body. When it becomes depleted and overloaded, your body bogs down and starts running in a compromised fashion—much like when your computer is overloaded. You don't notice it until out of nowhere your operating system starts to respond sluggishly, costing you time and frustration. It simply has too many demands and too little processing power. There's no need to scrap your computer—it's just time to reboot, perhaps defrag, and whatever else it takes to clear the slate and get it running at full operating speed.

Likewise, you need to regularly take a step back, recharge and reboot your body's systems. And once you do, you'll be stunned to discover just how sluggishly your system was operating.

BACK TO BALANCE WITH A LITTLE R&R AT BASE CAMP

In order to fulfill your potential in the 12 weeks that follow, it is in your best interest to begin your Transformation fully revitalized. And that's precisely what these 12 days of Base Camp are all about—helping you get ready to *start strong*.

Appropriately named after the camp where the essential and final preparations are made by those seeking to scale the world's highest summit—that of Mount Everest—Base Camp is a period of preparation. It's a time to rest, recover, rejuvenate, and recharge your body and mind. It's not a time of more, but of less. It's a time to relax the systems, not overwhelm them with new demands.

Getting back to balance begins with healing your body on the inside. When this happens, it's not unusual for your body to "super-compensate" by adding a small amount of muscle—for when you give it the chance to recover, it's likely to bounce back a little stronger. This may also lead to a slight drop in body fat percentage, just as Tom's client experienced.

It's not the numbers that are important here—it's the magic of setting the environment right for success, from the inside. In our attempt to focus on *doing* the right things, we often ignore our all-important physical state, which ultimately determines if the *right actions* produce the *right results*.

By now you may be feeling the draw to leap into your Transformation. Perhaps you're inspired to embrace the benefits of Focus Intensity Training or to simply get on to the promise of a new, stronger, leaner you. To feel this kind of passion at this point is terrific. But now is the time where you must show the patience to make the right step first—not the one that *looks* right, but the one that sets you up for success.

Whether you're new to this sort of a Transformation program, a veteran of another, or perhaps you're getting back to training after a layoff, the 12 days of Base Camp are the right way to begin.

Take these 12 days now to rejuvenate—enjoy them. Watch for the signs of your body returning to full strength: increased motivation, sleeping better, being free from sugar cravings. Even if you've been training for 20 years, you will find this period rejuvenating both mentally and physically. I realize this process might seem counterintuitive to you because it flies in the face of everything you know about getting things done and reaching goals. But I'm asking you to trust me on this; taking one small step back now will be a giant leap forward later.

Follow this simple guide and I promise that at the end of this brief 12-day Base Camp you will feel mentally and physically better than you have in years and be ready to get the most out of your *Strength for Life* Transformation. Feeling rested, recharged, and renewed at the end of your 12 days, you'll be popping out of bed full of vigor just like my son Nathaniel does every morning.

THE FULL SYSTEM REBOOT

FIVE RULES FOR THE 12 DAYS OF BASE CAMP

1. Eat "Lean, Clean, and Green."
2. Drink water in abundance.
3. Enjoy a minimum of seven hours restful sleep each night.
4. Flex your muscle of gratitude and positive focus daily.
5. Recharge with the Base Camp Training Plan.

REBOOT RULE NO. 1:
Eat Lean, Clean, and Green

How you fuel your body has an enormous impact on your state of strength and well-being. During these 12 days of Base Camp, your *only* dietary guideline is: *Eat Lean, Clean, and Green.* You will remove a number of foods from your diet completely to cleanse and balance your body.

Eating *lean* is enjoying an abundance of lean sources of protein like chicken breast, turkey, coldwater fish, lean beef, and egg whites. (I provide a food list of approved protein sources in this chapter.) Consuming protein at every meal will put you on the fast track to strength.

Eating *clean* means removing all forms of conventional fast food, heavily processed food, and other "junk" food from your diet. During this time, you'll consume no refined sugars. Twelve days away from refined sugars helps to stabilize your blood sugar and insulin levels and does wonders for your body on many levels.

Others on the do-not-consume food list include dairy products, breads, and alcohol—including the much revered red wine. It's only 12 days, and you'll be able to stock your bread box again soon enough. It's not that any of these foods are necessarily bad; it's that we're going to revive your body, and these are foods that can inhibit the system reboot.

Fresh fruits have natural sugar, therefore you are allowed to enjoy them. Similarly, high-quality whey protein, while technically dairy, is lactose-free and therefore permitted.

Eating *green* means if it's a vegetable, especially if it's green, eat it early and often. Enjoy the rediscovery of everything green during these next 12 days. Have a salad with breakfast and dip a carrot in a shot of wheat grass. Go green crazy. Enjoy your veggies without limits.

Base Camp Essentials

LEAN PROTEINS:	CARBS	FRUITS VEGGIES	HEALTHY FATS:	BEVERAGES
chicken*	yams	apples	unsalted nuts:	water
turkey*	brown rice	asparagus	almonds	green tea
fresh fish	old-fashioned	avocados	cashews	herbal tea
lean buffalo	oatmeal	bell peppers	pecans	
lean beef	whole-grain	berries (all kinds)	walnuts	in moderation:
egg whites	pasta	black beans		juices
tofu	quinoa	broccoli	olive oil	coffee
		brussels sprouts	avocados	
		cantaloupe	flaxseed	
		carrots		
		celery		
		cucumber		
		grapefruit		
		green beans		
		green peas		
		mushrooms		
		oranges		
		snap peas		
		spinach		
		tomatoes		
		yams		
		zucchini		
*Free-range, organic				

Nutrition Shakes:

Full Strength Premium Nutrition Shake is my performance fast food that's perfect first thing in the morning or for that midmorning or midafternoon meal. More on Full Strength in Chapter 10.

REBOOT RULE NO. 2:
Drink an Abundance of Water

Drink at least ten eight-ounce glasses of fresh and clean water daily to stay hydrated. For an athlete, a 1 percent drop in hydration can reduce performance output by as much as 20 percent. For the average person, dehydration increases the accumulation of toxins in the body, stunts metabolism, increases the risk of cancer, and accelerates the aging processes. In a dehydrated state, the mind and body do not operate at optimal levels.

Your body most effectively absorbs water in small amounts, so it's wise to drink it throughout the day. Water that is high-quality filtered or bottled at the source is best. You can enjoy fruit and vegetable juices; however, don't think that these can replace drinking water. Juice is a once-a-day type of thing at most. Drinking too much juice—especially fruit juice—will load you with sugar and calories. Avoid the consumption of "energy" or "sports" drinks, which are often laden with sugars that you don't need unless you are performing in an athletic event.

REBOOT RULE NO. 3:
Enjoy at Least Seven Hours of Restful Sleep Each Night

Restful sleep is a fundamental necessity for your well-being. Regardless of how busy you are, sleep is not optional. The quality and duration of your sleep has a direct impact on the levels of stress you experience and how well you cope.

Cortisol, the stress hormone, triggers both the breakdown of lean muscle and promotes the storage of fat. As you prepare yourself to build lean muscle, increase your strength, and burn fat, you must align your internal environment to support your goals. This means getting the sleep you require. In one study published in the *Journal of Sleep,* individuals who slept for only four hours produced cortisol levels on average 37 percent higher than those who got a full eight hours of sleep.

In Base Camp, I'm requesting you get seven to eight hours of sleep each night to keep your cortisol levels down and recovery up. Ideally this will be *restful* sleep, where you're not waking up frequently. Enjoy a low-key, winding-down period before going to bed to improve the quality of your sleep.

Writing Your Own Ticket to Freedom

Keep a 12-Day Food, Mood, and Energy Journal

Besides rejuvenating and priming your body for the Transformation ahead, Base Camp's Lean, Clean, and Green eating practice will help you develop an understanding of how food affects your energy levels and mood.

I've found that keeping a daily food journal is a useful practice (more on this in Chapter 10). Use a spiral notebook and track *everything* you eat on the left-hand side of a page and record how you felt (mood and energy) following each meal on the right-hand side.

By eating lean, clean, and green meals frequently and by keeping a journal throughout the day, you'll come to understand the relationship between what you eat and how you feel. By the end of Base Camp your awareness will be greatly tuned. By the end of your Transformation phase, you'll be in near perfect harmony with your body, to the point that you'll feel it when you eat something that tanks your energy, as an overdose of carbohydrates or high-fat foods can do.

This increased awareness of how food impacts your mood, energy levels, and performance is a giant leap toward freedom from dieting—where you freely choose the foods that are the best for you.

REBOOT RULE NO. 4:
Flex Your Muscle of Gratitude and Positive Focus Each Day

The thoughts that occupy your mind from moment to moment either elevate your energy and provide you with a sense of power and freedom or drain you, adding stress and bringing you down. It's that simple. Gratitude is like a muscle. Your ability to feel appreciation and find the positive in everything is strengthened through regular training, just like your muscles. That's why Base Camp includes a simple practice of expressing gratitude and appreciation each morning.

Once awake, find something—anything—for which you can quietly express gratitude. It could be the view outside your bedroom window, the sounds of the city coming to life, or your partner sleeping beside you. Just be thankful in the moment. Don't try to justify it—just feel it. No strings attached.

A great way to build this muscle of gratitude throughout the day is by reflecting on your appreciation for the food you enjoy. Once again, take a moment to be grateful for all that you have and all who are involved in you enjoying this food.

Finally, at the end of the day spend a few minutes reflecting on or even journaling (this is a great practice for life) about the three best things that happened for you during the day. Find your gratitude, note it, and let it soak in. This simple practice will have you seeing more and more of all that is good in this world. As Lou Tice, a highly respected educator and chairman of the Pacific Institute, says, "Your perception creates your reality, what you focus on becomes the world you create."

REBOOT RULE NO. 5:
Recharge with the Base Camp Training Plan

Forgo any form of intense training and follow only the Base Camp plan for these 12 days. Remember: This is a time to renew and recharge, to strengthen the connection between your body and mind. This might feel painfully simple, especially if you're a training veteran, but stay with the program, regardless.

You will train only three times a week: Mondays, Wednesdays, and Fridays. Your workouts begin with 10 minutes of light cardio work. Following this warm-up, you engage in a series of low-intensity body-weight movements.

You are going to do three sets of three different exercises. A "set" is a number of repetitions or movements of an exercise.

Give yourself enough time to catch your breath in between each set (about 30 seconds).

Again, this might look like a modest workout with basic exercises, which is exactly the point. Remember, the purpose of Base Camp training is not to tax you, but to rejuvenate and energize your body while you develop your mind–body connection. After the exercise descriptions following, I offer you an instruction on how to do a perfect push-up. This is a vivid example of the sort of form and focus you apply to every rep of every set during Base Camp.

STRENGTH FOR LIFE WORKOUT TRACKER

Base Camp: Mon/Wed/Fri **BASE CAMP TRAINING**

DATE _____ BASE CAMP DAY _____ START TIME _____ FINISH TIME _____

	SET	EXERCISE	TBS	PLANNED REPETITIONS	ACTUAL REPETITIONS
		Cardio Warm-Up: 10 Minutes			
UPPER BODY	1	Push-Ups (on knees if needed)		15–20 Reps	
	2		30	15–20 Reps	
	3		30	15–20 Reps	
LOWER BODY	4	Squats or Lunges	30	15–20 Reps	
	5		30	15–20 Reps	
	6		30	15–20 Reps	
CORE	7	Ab Crunches	30	12–15 Reps	
	8		30	12–15 Reps	
	9		30	12–15 Reps	

|TBS| = TIME *BEFORE* SET (Seconds)

NOTES

CARDIO WARM-UP

You can walk, jog, or bike, but if you find you're moving at a pace where you cannot hold a conversation, slow down. You're moving too fast.

PUSH-UPS

Starting Position: Start facing the floor while placing your hands beneath your shoulders approximately shoulder width apart. Your thumbs should be pointing toward each other while your fingers point straight ahead of you. Press up onto your toes, creating a straight line between your head, shoulders, hips, knees, and toes. Don't let your hips sag or rise up. If you find yourself breaking form, you may rest your knees on the ground, keeping the straight line between your knees, hips, shoulders, and head.

Start

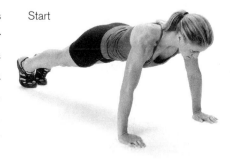

The Exercise: Slowly lower your body until your chest or chin is just about to touch the floor. Pause for a second and press yourself back up, stopping just before your arms are completely straight. Repeat.

Midpoint

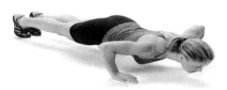

Sideview

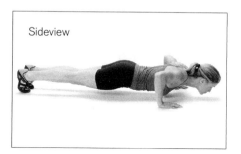

Finish

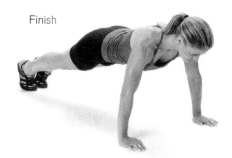

SQUAT

Starting Position: Stand with your feet parallel and slightly wider than shoulder width apart. Hold your arms out in front of you at shoulder height. You may choose to clasp your hands.

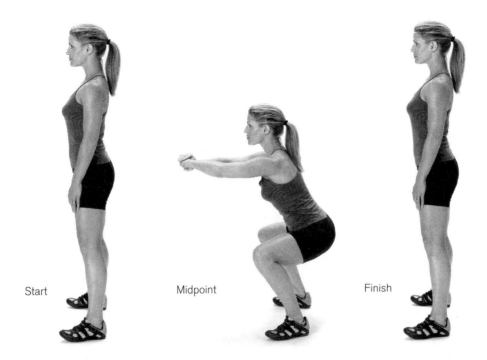

Start   Midpoint   Finish

The Exercise: While keeping your back flat and head upright, bend your legs at the knees and lower your hips as if you're sitting down into a chair. Continue to lower your hips until your thighs are parallel with the floor. Then slowly yet forcefully push down into the floor through your heels and toes, standing back up to the starting position. Inhale on the way down and exhale as you stand up.

ONE-LEGGED LUNGES (alternative to squats)

Starting Position: Stand with feet together, toes pointed forward. Keep your back straight, shoulders and hips squared, and chin up.

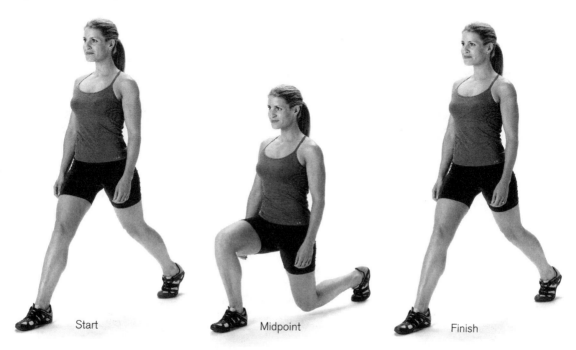

Start   Midpoint   Finish

The Exercise: Step forward with the right foot. While inhaling, bend at the knees, and lower the hips until the left knee is just a few inches off the floor and your front leg is at a 90-degree angle. Exhaling, push up and back with the right leg and bring your feet together, raising your body to the starting point. Complete all reps with your right leg before continuing to your left leg.

AB CRUNCH

Starting Position: Start by lying on your back with your knees bent and feet resting flat on the floor. Gently position your hands behind your head without locking your fingers.

Start

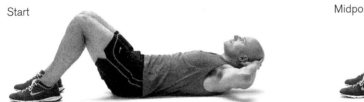

Midpoint

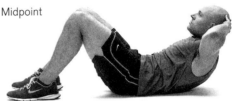

Finish

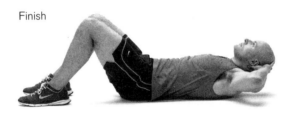

The Exercise: Slowly curl your body from your chest, lifting shoulders up and bringing your chest toward your knees until your upper back is off the floor. Avoid jerking or pulling your head up and do not sit all the way up. At the top of the movement contract your abs fully, having exhaled all of your air. Pause here for a two-second count, then slowly lower your torso back down, stopping just before your shoulder blades touch the floor. Repeat.

PUSH-UPS FROM THE INSIDE OUT

Begin by getting into a push-up position (if you need to do push-ups on your knees, that's okay). Breathing normally, check in with your body—running your awareness up from your feet, through your legs, into your midsection, and finally to the top of your head. You'll feel your toes on the ground, your hips locked, energy building in your upper body as you're supporting your weight, readying for the first push-up. Quickly set your intention: "I intend to complete 15 perfect, strong push-ups with total focus." This entire process should take 10 to 15 seconds.

Next, begin lowering your body toward the ground, feeling the stretch and stress, first in your chest muscles and moving out to your shoulders and triceps. As you lower on this rep, and all reps, you will breathe in—filling your lungs with a comfortable level of air. Keep it slow and steady as you go. When you reach the lowest point, your chest nearly touching the floor, make a slight pause before pressing back up. Don't lock and hold but ensure a full separation between the lowering and pressing back to top.

As you're pressing back up slowly and powerfully, your attention is focused deep within the muscles—you can feel your strength. Press the floor down with your hands, exhaling the air in your lungs with some force. Contract your chest, shoulders, and triceps with intensity through the entire range of motion. And on the way up, rather than simply pushing your hands straight down, try squeezing them together as if to slide your hands together. This will engage the chest and triceps more fully.

As you near the top position, stop just before your elbows fully lock. During each push-up, keep your cadence strong and smooth, not fast and jerky. Once you settle into a pace, hold it steady. If this feels too easy compared to the intense workouts you most enjoy, try taking it very slow—half speed or less—and that should help pick up the intensity.

You'll find that the combination of focusing on the quality of each rep with a steady cadence to be an entirely different experience than traditional rapid-fire push-ups.

In order to keep your cadence slow and steady, it may help to use a mantra like the one employed so effectively in *Body-for-LIFE*. If you choose to use this technique, try this rendition of the classic, "I am living at full strength." I prefer to focus on each rep and counting—and you can do this too once you've mastered the speed. In Chapter 11 I will share a powerful technique for counting each rep that will dial in your laserlike focus.

BASE CAMP SCHEDULE

Start Base Camp on a Monday and finish it the following Friday. Then take the weekend off before beginning the Transformation phase. Your calendar should look like this:

			BASE CAMP TRAINING			
MON	**TUES**	**WED**	**THUR**	**FRI**	**SAT**	**SUN**
DAY 1 TRAIN	DAY 2 OFF	DAY 3 TRAIN	DAY 4 OFF	DAY 5 TRAIN	DAY 6 OFF	DAY 7 OFF
DAY 8 TRAIN	DAY 9 OFF	DAY 10 TRAIN	DAY 11 OFF	DAY 12 TRAIN	X	X

Finish Strong: The Perfect 12 in a Row

NOTICE: READ THIS BEFORE YOU BEGIN BASE CAMP.

Before you begin Base Camp, know that there is one condition you must meet before you can move on to your Transformation Training Camp.

Here's the catch: These must be 12 consecutive, successful days. If you succumb to one food that's not part of the program, start over. If you fail to drink an abundance of water each day, start over. If you have one beer on Day 11, you start over. If you get six hours sleep one night, start over. If you miss a training session, you know what to do. I'm quite serious. Why? It's simple. You cannot successfully challenge your body until it's in a positive environment first, and that's the goal with Base Camp.

Don't cheat yourself. You're the judge and jury of your own success. You can pretend you made it or allow yourself a slip, but why cheat yourself? If you choose not to keep your commitment for these 12 short days, if you can't stay on track here and be honest with yourself, how do you feel about your odds of completing the challenge of Transformation?

Think of it this way: If you were climbing Mount Everest and you acted with disrespect for the challenge ahead while still at Base Camp, you would not be allowed to proceed, right? The same is true here: If you don't maintain the discipline to complete 12 consecutive days, as required, you'll just get to try it again, and again if need be, until you do prove your mettle and strength to begin the ascent.

I know this might sound harsh, but it's a simple rule that actually shows compassion. It embraces the fact that you do have what it takes to complete the 12 days—and the strength to enjoy an amazing Transformation, so I'll just keep waiting until you choose to step up and accept your greatness. And once you've done that, once you're willing to know you have what it takes, you've set yourself up for success in your Transformation. You'll be set to soar to new heights.

Plus, consider that at the end of this 12-day Base Camp you will be feeling better, stronger, and more motivated than you have in years. And then you will be fully ready to start your Transformation from strength.

Turn the page—and let your journey begin.

CHAPTER 6

Your Blueprint for Brilliance

You've read this far and chances are you're making your way through Base Camp, which begs the following questions: Why get in the best shape of your life now? What factors in your life are driving your Transformation?

As you progress through Base Camp, take this time to define your life at full strength. A life with strength is a life of purpose—in which you are inspired by the energy to achieve what matters most to you. Think deeply about the goals you want to accomplish during the 12-week program and the vision you'd like to create for the next 12 months. What will you accomplish for yourself, your family, and your community?

You will establish your vision prior to setting your Transformation goals, because your vision serves as the compass, your "true north." Your true north is a gripping narrative or picture of your life one year from today. It's not just the things you want, but also includes the feelings, energy, and emotions that bring your vision to life.

Together, an inspiring vision and clear goals serve as a blueprint for your lasting success— your choice to live a strong life, however *you* define it. It's the life you're most drawn to live into, a brilliant future that pulls you forward each day with great force.

By creating a vision and then setting specific goals to get you there, you take the power of the Transformation process far beyond the physical realm. You're not just increasing the effectiveness of your workouts, but also your ability to excel in life.

Your vision empowers your training, and your training empowers your vision.

NAVIGATING TO YOUR TRUE NORTH

As you sketch your vision, which you'll do momentarily, be sure to set aside some uninterrupted time. Place yourself in an environment that's free from distractions and allows you to have the focus and time you need to establish a clear vision for your life one year from today. Consider the elements that seem most compelling and meaningful: relationships, career, finances—so long as they're tied into the notion of living a life of strength and freedom. These factors are important for they are the tangible magnets that will draw you through the challenges that lay ahead.

This is your time to paint a vivid picture of your life. Dare to dream big. You're raising the bar for yourself and your life here. What does that life include? And how do you *feel* having achieved this vision?

Don't edit as you go along, let it be a free-flowing process. There are no right or wrong answers. I often find that people tend to focus solely on tangible rewards. Such visions include a new career, home, car, or dream vacation. All of these things are terrific, but don't forget to link them to *feelings*. It's ultimately the emotion that inspires you to move, to take action. Here are several examples:

- **I feel more energy than I have in years.**
- **My confidence is soaring; I feel like I can accomplish anything.**
- **I feel strong and powerful.**
- **I am clear, calm, and in control of my life.**
- **I feel productive, using my time effectively and efficiently.**

Use your journal or a blank sheet of paper for this exercise. If you prefer, write in this book; it will be rewarding to look back years from now and see how much you've achieved. Raise the bar and establish a vision that exceeds your know-how and even your current comfort zone. This way, you'll be challenged to grow and reach your next level of excellence.

Before you begin, please recite the following out loud:

> "I'm free to create my life exactly as I want it to be. There are no limitations. My life is now even more rewarding and satisfying. I'm filled with joy, gratitude, and energy now that these things are true."

Let your mind flow freely, capturing as many aspects of your vision as possible. These can be single words, short phrases, or incomplete sentences. Go for quantity. You might want to take several sessions to adequately complete this process.

Go.

My One-Year Vision Is:

_____

_____

_____

When you feel like you're ready to move on, review your ideas and write down the three to five most compelling, energizing elements. Note the feelings you associate with each, and condense them into one powerful, clear, concise vision.

My Most Compelling Elements Are:

1. _____

2. _____

3. _____

4. _____

5. _____

Note: If you're having trouble narrowing your list of ideas, it might help to eliminate those items that don't produce strong positive emotions. For instance, I enjoy playing golf, but I'm not especially passionate about it. Thus, being a scratch golfer isn't going to inspire me. I won't be able to create the energy to fulfill this part of my vision. On the other hand, _you_ might be an avid golfer who not only loves the game but sees it translate into greater business opportunities and a higher quality of life. Being a scratch golfer definitely would be part of a compelling vision for you. One thing is certain, if you fail to define your life, life will define you.

THE POWER OF GOALS

With your vision in mind, it's time to set your goals for your Transformation. Goals are the defined, measurable outcomes you intend to achieve in a given period of time, in this case over the course of the next 12 weeks. Goals are your markers along the path of life moving you toward your vision.

Too often people see vision and goals as one and the same. Goals need to be separate, albeit supportive, of the vision and must be specific, challenging, and meaningful, not vague wishes or fleeting desires. Effective goal setting is one of the secrets to a life of success.

Part of the reason people don't set goals is because it's easy to fail, even though there is nothing more empowering and rewarding than setting and achieving a lofty goal. So why then do we sometimes fail to reach our goals? How can something we so clearly desired just seem to fade away?

The answer lies in physics, the fundamental laws that govern the universe. Understanding this will enlighten and empower you to achieve your goals with greater consistency, improved determination, and to do so faster than ever before.

One of the most well-known and important laws of physics is Newton's Law of Universal Gravitation. This nearly 400-year-old law states: "Every object in the universe attracts every other object, with a force that depends on the object's mass and distance between them."

A planet has a certain mass—the greater the mass, the stronger the gravitational pull. Mass is only part of the equation; the other part is the *distance* between the two objects. The relationship or tension between the two is known as gravity.

Think of goals as if they were objects, like planets. They have a mass—the more meaningful and important the goal, the larger its "mass." Goals also have a distance, the time between setting the goal and when you plan to achieve it. The further away the goal is in time, the less pull it has, regardless of importance.

Achieving your goals is due in large part to uniting the right balance of meaning and significance (mass) with the right time frame (distance) to create the necessary force of attraction (gravitational pull).

For example, you might want to sculpt your best body, and this might be a clearly defined goal with great *mass*—or importance—to you. But if the distance between you and the achievement of the goal, as you define it, is too great, it will not pull you forward strong enough or long enough to bring you to your goal. The *Strength for Life* program is intelligently segmented into three distinct measurable phases: 12 days, 12 weeks, 12 months to generate the pull necessary to deliver you to your goals.

SETTING GOALS

Numerous studies have made a link between putting your goals on paper and achieving them. Setting goals brings them into focus and transfers them from your head into action. It's been my experience that goals not written down simply are not achieved; they're just ideas or wishes.

To achieve goals, you must eliminate words such as "hopefully" and "maybe" and "can't" from your thinking. It's not enough to say, "I want to get in shape." This is the traditional New Year's resolution that has no power, no direction behind it. It's not specific. It's not a goal, but a vague wish.

Instead, if you want to go from a size 14 to a size 8 or from a 38-inch waist to a 34-inch waist within 12 weeks, those are specific and measurable. It makes a considerable difference. Be ambitious, but realistic. What can you accomplish in 12 weeks?

It helps to have a specific time line. I've found there's nothing more effective for whipping me into shape than a deadline of an upcoming vacation or photo shoot. A deadline creates that immediate sense of urgency and helps to prioritize daily activities.

I want you to set four goals for the next 12 weeks. The first two are *physical* goals as judged by objective measurements. These can be quantified, such as losing ten pounds of fat, gaining three pounds of muscle, losing two inches off your waistline, lowering your cholesterol, decreasing blood pressure, or reducing your resting heart rate.

The next two goals focus on your *inner* strength. These are subjectively measured and not as easy to quantify, but are no less important. After all, self-improvement is not just physical. These are mental and emotional-based goals.

Focus on improving your outlook, attitude, mood, and knowledge base. Think of how you deal with stress, interact with loved ones and co-workers, or deal with adversity. Consider making goals of improving in some of these areas. For example, you could improve your relationship with someone who holds a significant amount of importance in your life. Or perhaps you're looking to advance your career or personal growth. You could set a goal of reading a certain number of books, taking new courses, or hiring a professional coach to support and challenge you.

List your four goals:

Physical Goal 1:

Physical Goal 2:

Inner Strength Goal 1:

Inner Strength Goal 2:

_____

You will learn how to leverage these goals effectively as part of the daily and weekly practice I will help you establish in the next chapter.

Case Study

James
37 years old
5'11"
188 pounds Pre-Transformation
Married, three children (ages 5, 8, 12)
177 pounds Post-Transformation

In recent years my friend James spent long hours at his office, no longer worked out regularly, and was eating poorly: skipping breakfast, drinking sodas throughout the day, and using the drive-through almost daily for lunch. As a result he had packed on about 15 extra pounds.

Like a lot of driven professionals, James sought more responsibility, a better salary, and an executive level position at his company.

While in Base Camp, James defined his vision as follows:

> I have the energy I did ten years ago. I am more efficient and productive at my job now, demonstrating greater leadership, taking on more responsibility. My efforts have been rewarded through a salary increase, and a promotion. By being more efficient, I'm spending less time at work and better quality time with the kids. Next month we're taking an eight-day vacation to Maui, where I'll squeeze in a round of golf. I'm maintaining the strength and vitality I gained in my Transformation and I'm feeling great.

Next, James set physical, emotional, and mental goals that served as a support structure for his vision. He realized that if he wanted to live at full strength and lose excess weight, he needed to gain energy and stamina while swapping body fat for lean muscle. _continued on next page_

From an emotional standpoint, James knew that he let himself get dragged down by problems at work. He'd come home deflated, with little energy for his family. He recognized that his physical Transformation would give him more energy, allow him to work more efficiently, and not feel constantly run-down.

Finally, James looked at things from a mental standpoint. He realized that he needed to increase his knowledge and improve his management skills to attain his promotion.

Here's a look at James's 12-week goals:

> **PHYSICAL GOALS:** I will lose 15 pounds of fat, gain 4 pounds of lean muscle, and lose 2 inches around my waist by April 10th and am enjoying high energy and soaring confidence.
>
> **MENTAL/EMOTIONAL GOALS:** I will bring positive energy to share with my wife and children. We'll enjoy one family activity each week. I'll read two leadership books and hire a business coach to strengthen my career by April 10th.

Not a bad start, James. He's broken down his vision into quantifiable goals such as losing 15 pounds, gaining four pounds of lean muscle, and reading two books on leadership. He recognizes that in order to contribute more to his family, friends, and community, he must feel confident and energetic. He's thought beyond his own immediate achievements by connecting his goals to something bigger than himself—his family.

James initially was skeptical about reaching his goals and vision. Then a funny thing happened. Within days of leaving Base Camp, he began to feel that confidence and energy.

He was following through on the nutrition and exercise program we'll discuss in more detail in the coming chapters, along with his goal of reading one book every six weeks on leadership. James started offering more insight and advice to coworkers. As the weeks went by he was amazed at his progress.

James began losing fat and gaining muscle. He could chart his progress not only by his weekly measurements, but also by how his clothes felt; soon needing some new items in his wardrobe. His family and coworkers marveled at his Transformation. But of even greater value to James was how he felt about himself and what he was accomplishing.

After 12 weeks he had transformed his body, dropping close to 17 pounds of fat and adding 6 pounds of lean muscle. He had more energy, made more time for his family, and though he didn't yet have a title at work that reflected the executive title he sought, he felt confident he was moving in the right direction.

CHAPTER 7

Progress Made Is Progress Measured

Imagine for a moment that you're on a road trip to sunny Southern California. Your car is packed and fueled, tunes jamming, and you're heading off on your adventure. Your destination is clear, your goal defined. Everything's going great until four or five hours into the trip when your energy fades, along with the vision of the beaches, giving way to boredom and fatigue. But you'll get there, soon enough. No problem.

A few hours later doubt begins to creep in and the questions start. Do you have enough gas? What about money? You've got no map, and as if that weren't bad enough, you realize that the odometer on your car is busted. You're tired, unsure, and can't tell how long you've been on the road.

At what point do you turn back? When do you give up? How do you continue when you're not sure where you are along the course? Without road markers to measure the distance covered, you're essentially lost. Even a goal becomes nothing more than a wish.

This is exactly the way most people approach their fitness goals. They get their eyes set on the prize, bursting with desire and motivation. All psyched up, they merge onto the nearest "fitness expressway," only to wind up as a roadside casualty, fizzling out as rapidly as they jumped in.

The simple practice of relentlessly tracking and measuring your progress is the most effective way to maintain your course and produce your best results. It's vital to your Transformation success. Progress made is progress measured.

Now, imagine you're on the same trip, but this time with a map, an odometer, a watch, etc.

With every click of the mile, with every mark in time, you're making progress and feeling the achievement.

Achieving results builds confidence, reinforcing your ability to achieve again and again; you soon will come to expect results (as opposed to wishing and hoping) throughout your Transformation, as well as in other areas of your life.

YOUR TRANSFORMATION MEASUREMENTS AND PHOTOGRAPHS

At the beginning of your Transformation phase and continuing throughout the 12 weeks, you will be tracking your progress with the help of photographs and statistical measurements. First up, you will take your *before* measurements, barometers of your current, pre-Transformation physical condition. You will compare these against your post-Transformation results. Some of these can be done in-home, while your preferred health care professional best handles others.

Here are a few suggestions if you would like to capture some of these measurements yourself. Use skin calipers to measure your body fat percentage. To measure resting heart rate, place

TRANSFORMATION MEASUREMENTS

PRE-TRANSFORMATION	MEASUREMENT	POST-TRANSFORMATION
	DATE	
	WEIGHT	
	BODY FAT %	
	RESTING HEART RATE	
	BLOOD PRESSURE	
	CHOLESTEROL	
	CORONARY RISK RATIO*	
	OTHER:	
	OTHER:	

*Coronary Risk Ratio, often referred to as CRR, is your HDL/LDL and is recognized as an important contributing factor to the cause or prevention of heart disease.

your index and middle fingers together on the opposite wrist, about a half inch on the inside of the joint; when you find a pulse, count the number of beats you feel within a one-minute period, or use an exercise heart rate monitor.

Tracking Your Progress: Weekly

Measuring where you've come from is essential to improving your confidence, sustaining momentum, and tracking where you're going. You do this by staying focused on the distance covered, not the distance to go. In the previous example, if you have 1,000 miles to go on your road trip, it is much more rewarding to celebrate the distance already covered. This positive focus feeds you, where the focus on what is yet to be covered can be frustrating or at times even demoralizing.

If your goal is to lose, say, 12 pounds, celebrate the first 2 pounds lost, then the next 2, rather than focusing on the 8 still to go.

Photographs: Seeing Your Progress

Starting with Day One, take weekly photos of yourself: front, back, and from each profile. Shoot the photos in the same position and location, wearing the same shorts or bathing suit each time. At the end of 12 weeks, you'll be able to put together a stack of photos and literally see yourself transforming.

Physical Measurements

Use a cloth tape measure to help track your changes. Choose at least two of the following measurements that will enable you to objectively track your progress week to week: Waistline, Hips, Thighs, Chest, Arms, Weight, and Body Fat. Note: If you track weight, you may actually see an increase in your first several measurements; not necessarily a cause for concern if you're following the program as designed. This increase is most likely due to a gain in lean muscle, which will ultimately help you burn fat.

RECONNECT WITH YOUR TRANSFORMATION GOALS

Having taken your photographs and recorded your physical measurements pre-Transformation, it's time to revisit your goals. I'd like you to rewrite them as affirmations, using the present tense. Affirmations can be valuable in managing your mood, building self-confidence, and helping you focus. Feeding your mind with positive messages is just as important as feeding your body with energy-producing foods.

FRONT: PRE-TRANSFORMATION

PLACE YOUR
IMAGE HERE

BACK: PRE-TRANSFORMATION

PLACE YOUR
IMAGE HERE

FRONT: POST-TRANSFORMATION

PLACE YOUR
IMAGE HERE

BACK: POST-TRANSFORMATION

PLACE YOUR
IMAGE HERE

RIGHT PROFILE: PRE-TRANSFORMATION

PLACE YOUR
IMAGE HERE

LEFT PROFILE: PRE-TRANSFORMATION

PLACE YOUR
IMAGE HERE

RIGHT PROFILE: POST-TRANSFORMATION

PLACE YOUR
IMAGE HERE

LEFT PROFILE: POST-TRANSFORMATION

PLACE YOUR
IMAGE HERE

TRANSFORMATION GOALS

WEEK	GOAL #1: _____	GOAL #2: _____	GOAL #3 (OPTIONAL): _____	GOAL #4 (OPTIONAL): _____
1				
2				
3				
4				
5				
6				
7				
8				
9				
10				
11				
12				
PROGRESS*				

*Progress is determined by the difference between Week 1 and Week 12 measurements.

Examples:

Physical Goal 1: "I lost 12 pounds of fat."

Physical Goal 2: "I gained 4 pounds of lean muscle."

Inner Strength Goal 1: "I've read two books on self-improvement and completed an advanced leadership seminar."

Inner Strength Goal 2: "I feel more confident at work and I step boldly into leadership opportunities."

REPLACE HABITS WITH RITUALS

People tend to talk in terms of "good habits" and "bad habits," but I prefer to think in terms of rituals and habits. Think about it. The difference between rituals and habits is that you choose to do rituals with awareness and intention. People tend to admire rituals. Whenever you hear someone say, "She has a habit of . . ." the thing that comes next is rarely positive.

What are the habits that undermine your progress and success? Could it be mindless eating in front of the television? Do you have a habit of failing to schedule your training? Do you have the habit of letting "things" compromise your free time?

In order to accomplish your 12-week goals, and ultimately make progress toward your vision, it's necessary to establish a daily pattern of positive actions—new rituals that generate progress every day. You'll do this through a "morning strength ritual" and an "evening reflection."

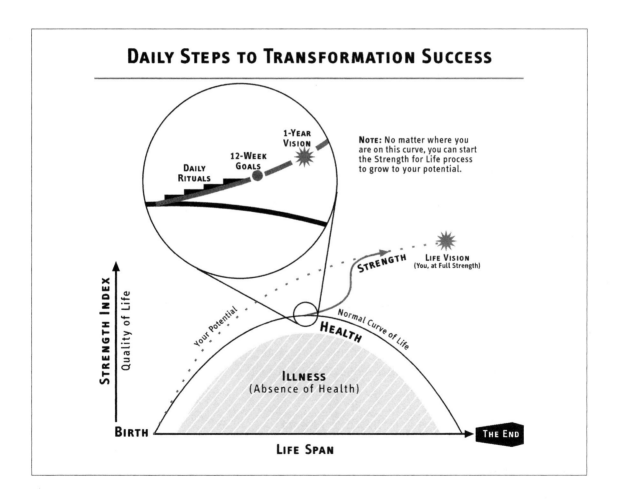

In the morning you will project, plan, and set your course for the day. In the evening you'll reflect back, evaluate, and make critical course corrections. You'll be watching the "game film," so to speak, reviewing what worked, evaluating what didn't, and planning to make the appropriate changes in tomorrow's game.

These rituals should take about five minutes first thing in the morning, to start your day strong, and another five minutes to close your day, with the intention to stay on course and continually improve daily.

MORNING STRENGTH RITUAL

I know. You already have a morning ritual. It consists of some combination of training, breakfast (more about this in Chapter 10), showering, personal grooming, and getting the kids off to school.

Before you do any of that, however, I want you to perform a brief morning strength ritual that will propel you through the day and keep you on track throughout the program. It will be the first thing you do when you awaken during your upcoming 12-week Transformation.

Step One: Appreciate Something upon Waking

As discussed in Chapter 5, the act of appreciating is like a muscle. If it's not used, it goes away. Often we focus on the challenges and tasks that lie ahead. Instead of diving into the day's challenges, take a moment and appreciate something in your life. It can be the sight of your significant other still sleeping, an opportunity to wake up the kids, or the view of a sunrise. Whatever you choose, spend a moment appreciating it to set you in the right frame of mind for the day.

Step Two: Review Your Vision and Goals

Next, connect with your vision and briefly review your goals now that they are written as affirmations. Keep this book close by, with the vision and goal pages marked for easy reference. Make a photocopy of them or rewrite your vision and goals in a journal. Whatever you do, make sure these are easily accessible.

Step Three: Review Your Key Daily Action Items

Before you start your day, review your daily opportunities for strength, which you keep on a piece of paper or in a journal at your bedside.

1. Complete my morning strength ritual.

2. Eat five balanced meals today.

3. Train (assuming it is not an off day).

4. Maintain a positive, optimistic outlook.

5. Complete my evening reflection.

6. Sleep seven to eight hours.

EVENING REFLECTION

One of the greatest challenges in any fitness and nutrition regimen is sticking with the program. Life tends to get in the way. When you're living at strength, however, you're making a point to follow through on your goals and vision.

The Evening Reflection is the last thing you do before laying your head on the pillow. The mind is very receptive before you go to sleep, and you want to reinforce everything you're accomplishing before drifting off.

Before you turn off the lights, review your daily opportunities for strength. Ask yourself, did I:

1. Sleep seven to eight hours last night?

2. Complete my morning strength ritual?

3. Eat five balanced meals today?

4. Train (assuming it was not an off day)?

5. Maintain a positive, optimistic outlook?

6. Complete my evening reflection?

Celebrate what you accomplished. Be thankful for it. Don't be afraid to make a "course correction" to ensure your daily progress.

The last thing you should do before turning out the lights is reread your vision.

Are you going to score 100 percent every day? Probably not, and that's okay. As you'll come to know, the closer you get to your goal, the more it draws you in; success feeds success. It's the gravitational pull. Once you get into a rhythm, progress is hard to stop. You achieve big visions by doing the little things every day with a positive mind-set.

If you're someone who keeps a journal, include your experiences in your entries. If you've never kept a journal, this might be a good time to start. A journal is a powerful way to "course correct," because it allows you to see a pattern of what's working effectively for you and what is not.

STRENGTH FOR LIFE **TRANSFORMATION COMMITMENT**

I, _____, commit to working diligently and consistently over the next 12 weeks to accomplish my goals and improve the overall strength I bring to my life.

Signature: _____

Date: _____

Transformation Training Camp: 12 Weeks That Will Change Your Life

We acquire the strength
we have overcome.
—RALPH WALDO EMERSON

CHAPTER 8

Forging Your Strength for Life

It's your time to begin the noble climb from out of the *ordinary* to the heights of *extraordinary.* Having completed your preparation in the 12 days of Base Camp, you are now ready to enter the 12 weeks of Transformation.

Your body is an amazingly adaptive machine. Ask it to be stronger, and stronger you will be. Challenge it to go further, and further you will go. Coax it to be more limber, and more limber you will be. Allow it to mold into the seat of a recliner and—you got it—a recliner seat it will become. Stretch it, push it, pull it; your body is like cellular Play-Doh waiting for you to be the sculptor.

In this lifetime you will experience no greater direct influence on your quality of life than in the strengthening of your body and mind. By accepting this opportunity to enjoy abundant energy, release pounds, erase years, and completely reshape your body, you're in control. For some, this may mean taking your body *back* to a previous high point. For others, it's pushing to a new summit and enjoying a physical peak beyond any previously known.

Think of the next 12 weeks as your *Training Camp* for a strong life. For athletes, training camp is a focused, intensive period of time specifically designed to transform from their off-season condition to their peak of in-season performance, physically and mentally. I can find no more accurate description of what the 12 weeks ahead will be for you.

WHY 12 WEEKS?

The *Strength for Life* Training Camp is an intensive period of strengthening your body *and* mind—the culmination of everything I've learned about sensible, effective training and nutrition over the course of decades.

One of the most oft-asked questions I receive is, "Why 12 weeks?"

Twelve weeks is nearly magical. It's long enough to make significant life changes and short enough that you can make it to the end. In some early Transformation programs eight weeks was tried, and it simply did not prove to be as effective as 12 for numerous reasons. But the strongest argument for 12 over 8—or even 10—is that the body seems to adjust in stages, sort of ratcheting itself up in steps. And the final four weeks has been shown to be the most fertile time for results. The body really starts kicking into a new gear in this last month—when, often, nearly fifty percent of the gains come.

Unfortunately, it's also the case that after a period of adapting, as your body does over the final four weeks, it's bound to hit a wall—which frequently occurs beyond 12 weeks. You get a little greedy and then the wheels of progress come off. So it's worth reminding yourself that you have 12 weeks to make your Transformation count—not 14 and not 16, but 12.

Transformations follow a reasonably predictable pattern of elevation with four distinct stages. While by no means precise, the pattern of stages does follow along fairly closely with 21-day intervals. I find that breaking the 12 weeks into four 21-day stages is helpful in maintaining focus and managing expectations. Your experience will be unique, but generally speaking, you will encounter each of these stages.

Stage One: Days 1 through 21

This stage is about momentum—aligning the numerous forces and factors in your favor. Think of your ascent as if it were a rocket taking off. It's the initial thousand feet that require the largest percentage of boost and fuel for your breaking out of the grips of gravity. Similarly, these few weeks will be both challenging and absolutely critical to reaching your full stride. This is a time to align your practice, creating your rhythm and rituals of training and nutrition. At times you may "not be feeling it," you might focus on the wrong things and even experience doubt. This stage can feel like more work than the following stages. Take it *one day* at a time, for 21 days in a row.

Stage Two: Days 22 through 42

At the Week Three milestone, plus or minus a few days, it's common that people express some frustration or concern. They just aren't feeling or seeing results yet. Don't worry, hang on. Any doubts will be resolved as you're greeted by your first noteworthy felt-sense breakthrough. When you've established a good rhythm, doing all the right things, your body will resist change for a while and then suddenly start working with you. This reward is usually boost enough to finish this 21-day sprint strong.

Stage Three: Days 43 through 63

As you enter into your third set of 21 days, know that at this stage you will experience a slight plateau. Bolstered by the first spurt of results, you can get a little spoiled—and that's when things slow a little. Now is your time to double-check your practices, make sure you're reaching training peaks, and hone your nutrition in preparation for the home stretch.

Stage Four: Days 64 through 84

In this final sprint, the stretch run, expect to question if you set your goals high enough. When a few weeks earlier you were filled with doubt, suddenly it's as if the force is with you. It's not uncommon for this last 21 days to produce the most rewarding measurable results.

BEYOND THE BODY

Your Transformation to your best body and life will not be achieved through long arduous hours, extreme training, complex exercises, amazing feats of strength, or a miracle diet. Instead, you will engage in a fully integrated training program that will strengthen and condition your mind, heart, and body; along with a sound nutrition strategy for significant and lasting change in your shape, strength, stamina, and overall state of well-being.

Proper nutrition is absolutely key to your success, and given that it's at least five times as likely to derail your progress, the nutrition practice precedes training in this section of the book. The goal is to feed your success with the right foods for strength.

As you indulge in the *Strength for Life* Training Camp, you may find it simple, but please don't confuse that with being one-dimensional. If you've been through a Transformation, you'll be familiar with the exercises. If you haven't seen the inside of a gym since junior high PE class, that's okay too. Complete descriptions are provided in Appendix D.

Unless you've nurtured a lifetime of inactivity, you will not find the amount of work or the duration of training sessions beyond your capacity. The daily time requirements should not be a stress to those with even the most hectic of schedules. In fact, I'd venture to say you'll find yourself capable of accomplishing more each day with your new energy.

Even if you've been training for more than 20 years, like me, and are set in your training knowledge, you might find there's a refreshing vibrancy that comes when you focus your training on "what really matters." If you're concerned that the workouts are too condensed, I invite you to step up your training intensity a notch or two and squeeze more out of each rep. You may be surprised how quickly muscle can be activated when you bring 100 percent of your concentration to training. Take these 12 weeks to deeply engage and embrace the Focus Intensity Training practice—and bring your mind along. Your strength will surely follow.

A WARNING BEFORE YOU CLIMB

While contemplating your dedication to the endeavor ahead, take a moment to review the goals you've established for the 12 weeks. As you read them, feel into your future. Are your goals strong? Powerful? Do you have a deeper meaning connected to the physical goals? In other words, does the new body you've defined have a clearly defined emotional meaning or impact?

If your goals are vague or lacking deep meaning, you may be reluctant—feel hesitant to engage with your Transformation. If so, take the opportunity to refine your goals with greater intention, clarity, and purpose. It's vital that you discover *that which lights your fire*. Focus on it and set yourself on a course for greatness. Do not wait for the "right time"—do it now, take advantage of the two-day break in between the close of Base Camp and Training Camp.

On the other hand, if you've done top-notch goal work already and your goals are clear, strong, and empowering, expect to feel drawn into the program with eagerness. Rather than seeing the schedules and details as what you "must do" or an obligation, see them as your "how to" road map to success.

While the *Strength for Life* Transformation Training Camp is a one-size-fits-all regimen, your destination—what you do with it—is as unique as you are. There is only one *you,* and thus one path that is *yours*. You can be as strong and fit as you choose.

THE JOY OF STRENGTH

That brings me to one of the success pillars supporting the *Strength for Life* Transformation. While this program may be more *effective* and *efficient* than any fitness transformation program you can find today, the real gift is that it embodies my passion and love for training and is designed to bring the joy of training to you.

It is now time for *action*—and this is where it gets to be fun. Here you'll find the tools, step-by-step instructions, and tips for success. You've already created your blueprint—only you can choose to bring it to life. Keep in mind that you will inhabit each moment of each day in the structure *you* create.

PACKING FOR SUCCESS

Approach the next 12 weeks as you would a great life adventure. Enter with an open mind and a light spirit—and seek to enlighten both. Give this all that you have, for in the final analysis this is but a brief period of time. You will be a stronger person in nearly every way for having done it.

It may help you stay on course to know that this Training Camp for Transformation is a phase. It is not required that you live this way each day for the rest of your life. You will choose how to live your life transformed in the final section of the book, Week 13 and Beyond.

One more word of advice before you begin: You will benefit from giving your training attire and cooking "gear" some much deserved attention, for they are both important components of your Transformation. I'll help you prep your kitchen for Transformation in Chapter 10. Right now I encourage you to treat yourself to some training attire worthy of your intention and your new body. This may seem like a small thing, but it's not at all. I believe that just as a beautiful, properly fitting suit or stunning dress can establish your state for a social event, your training clothes can set the stage for your Transformation.

Your clothing should be comfortable, form-fitting while not tight—preferably shorts or mid-length pants and a top. For comfort I find the quality cotton in fine yoga clothing to be splendid. I urge you to invest in a comfortable, supportive, and appropriately cool pair of shoes that will carry you well for the next 12 weeks. Please trash any old gym rags if you've got them. I don't want to see you in any old ripped up T-shirt or vertically striped tights. Just don't do it—it's not good for anyone involved.

Finally, expect to be challenged during these next 12 weeks, as life may conspire against you. Yes, that's right. Things will unexpectedly arise, so don't forget to pack your strength. Be prepared and stay your course.

Let the ascent begin.

CHAPTER 9

Eat to Live

The alluring aroma of fresh baked bread, the sizzling of a New York strip on the grill, the sparkling crispness of a tree-fresh Gala apple; food is magnificent, delectable, provocative, and powerful—one of life's finest pleasures. I enjoy food, all sorts of foods.

Food is quite literally fuel for life. Next to water, air, and the sun, nothing is more important to your life than the nutrition that food provides.

We must *eat to live*.

Unfortunately, more and more people have it backward. Rather than *eat to live,* they *live to eat*. Instead of food being in service of life, it becomes a center of life, a source of "happiness." As a result of this cultural misadaptation, the very thing that sustains life is taking it.

For all of food's impact in our lives, we often treat it with disrespect. We take it for granted, use it recklessly, and abuse it foolishly, all to our detriment. Rarely do we give food the attention it warrants. From this day forward I suggest you begin treating food with the respect you would give a loaded gun. While a gun is a more immediate threat, it has but a fraction of the impact food has on your life.

It's a given that anything with such immense power for enhancing your life also has the power to destroy. Which one it does is up to you; food can *elevate* and create you strong, or it can debilitate, handicap, and leave you weak.

Relax. I'm not suggesting another torturous diet, which for most people is little more than a draining period of deprivation doomed to failure. Your body knows what it needs to thrive, and it strives to supply the right balance of nutrients. Where diets fall short is by leading you to believe that you can somehow deny your body's natural desire for nourishment, which is intended to keep you living healthy and strong. This is the wrong approach, well intended in most cases but hopelessly misdirected—and certainly not the path to greater freedom, energy, and strength.

My wish for you is to enjoy each day the vibrant energy and strength that flows through you when you *nourish* your body and mind. Nourishment is the ultimate purpose of food—it means "the sustenance required to live, grow, and remain fit." Within these pages I will show you how to consistently eat in a way that elevates your mind, energizes your body, and transforms your life; and how to do so freely because you want to, not because you have to.

BE YOUR OWN SUPERHERO

Eating is a necessity, but *what* you eat is ultimately your choice. Remarkably, most people go a lifetime without learning even the basics of proper nutrition. They see food and reactively eat it. While I'm sure you'd agree that the resistance and discipline of dieting can be a tremendous effort, learning to bring your "higher mind" into your eating can be nothing less than heroic. But make no mistake, it's the path to a lifetime of nutritional freedom. No special powers or capes necessary.

When it comes to making the intelligent, empowering choices about what to eat and what not to eat, I choose life; which is to say I eat to live rather than live to eat. This means I'm free to choose *nourishment* over *food cravings*.

How I eat is the result of practiced awareness—a developed strength. You might call it a *conscious eating* practice. Think about how Tiger Woods swings a golf club: his mind clear and focused, he's not *thinking* about his swing. It's effortless. He's swinging the club the way he knows, the way he's rehearsed it a million times.

Often when I'm out to lunch with new friends or business associates, the food will arrive and someone will ask me, "How do you do it?"

"Do what?" I ask.

"Eat with such amazing discipline," they reply.

I usually offer a brief explanation: When I eat, I focus on high-quality lean protein and build the meal from there. I'll ask for substitutions as necessary, but for the most part I can find something that will work. I order from the same menu my friends use. It's the way I interpret it that is different. I see each meal as servings of protein, carbohydrates, and vegetables, and this helps me consistently choose food that is great for me.

When the meal arrives, I eat some of the protein first because protein slows the absorption

Dieting's Dirty Little Secret

Research into the success rate of diets has confirmed more than 95 percent of all dieters return to their original weight and then some—gaining on average of another ten pounds.

The authentic need for nourishing food that originates from your body can become distorted like an image through a dirty camera lens. If this happens before hunger enters your awareness, the life-supporting need for vital nutrients morphs into intense cravings and an insatiable appetite, usually for foods that are anything but life-enhancing.

As a result of this "dirty lens," over time your body becomes as distorted as the image you receive. And as long as this goes unchanged, you will continue eating the wrong foods, in the wrong amounts; damaging your body, draining your energy, and destroying your strength.

> ## The Four "D"s of Diets
>
> *Diets typically...*
>
> ☐ **D**rain energy and your life
>
> ☐ **D**eceive you with hope
>
> ☐ **D**eny your freedom
>
> ☐ Require extraordinary **D**iscipline

Diets try to combat cravings, but your subconscious mind does not distinguish this distorted message (craving) from an original authentic need for life-supporting nutrition. By denying the body's wish for nutrition, deep inside you're in opposition to your own life. This is why a restrictive diet can suddenly trigger the battle for survival: One minute you're bragging about the five pounds you've lost—the next minute you're in a life-and-death struggle with a doughnut!

Why take on this battle when by simply clearing off the dirty lens you can eliminate the distortion and embrace a life-enhancing relationship with food? This means getting in tune with your body's *true* need for the energy and vital nutrients in food. By developing your *Nutritional Awareness* you will enjoy a positive relationship with food and support your body's wisdom, which keeps you living strong.

of carbs into my body, meaning longer-lasting energy, greater satiety, and less fat storage. I'll eat the veggies and then some of the carbs, typically less than served. Many restaurants love to heap on carbs, serving you several times more than what you need, so it's your job to know what a portion is (I'll provide assistance in Nutritional Strategies in Chapter 10). Eating this way is ultimately not an act of great discipline—it's effortless. And from what I've been able to confirm, it's a skill much easier to master than a golf swing.

Before you can become a master, you must first know the rules of the game—the ins and outs—the art of eating. In Appendix B you'll find a list of foods that can elevate your performance. In the next chapter I'll present some basic, easy-to-follow guidelines for meals, along with tips on timing and eating patterns, portion sizes, and so forth. All very sound, helpful, and important tools for your Transformation. But as you will discover, it's not the dos and don'ts that will set you free. Rather, it's an entirely new way of relating to food that holds the key to learning how to eat to live.

A WHOLE NEW WAY TO THINK ABOUT NUTRITION

There are two distinct ways of relating to food. The more dominant way is to see food as a source of immediate gratification. This begins the moment you become aware of *cravings,* or hunger, and continues until the moment of *consumption.*

Food cravings arise between your ears. It's the satisfaction we hunger for, the good feeling that comes when we finally silence the emptiness. And there are few places where one can fill a void quicker than with food. When you're eating that sweet snack, you may think you're quieting the craving, but you're actually *feeding* it. As it turns out, the more one reacts to and feeds cravings, the stronger the cravings become and the more power they have.

When you eat like this—in reaction to cravings—you have what I call a *Cravings to Consumption* relationship with food. You have a craving that may be in part physical. You promptly hone in on something "good" to eat that will calm the craving, and after you consume the food, it's all over until next time.

If this sounds familiar, don't take it too hard—no one is immune. Few can say they've never allowed a craving to rule. For some it's now and then, but for others it's the predominant mode of eating.

When you're ruled by a craving, your focus on food ends when you eat. You go back to what you were doing before being so rudely interrupted by your hunger. The idea that your attention on nutrition ends right after you eat makes as much sense as a quarterback ignoring what hap-

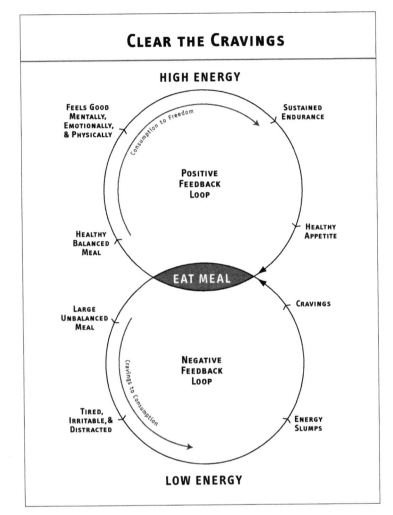

CLEAR THE CRAVINGS

HIGH ENERGY

FEELS GOOD
MENTALLY,
EMOTIONALLY,
& PHYSICALLY

SUSTAINED
ENDURANCE

Consumption to Freedom

POSITIVE
FEEDBACK
LOOP

HEALTHY
BALANCED
MEAL

HEALTHY
APPETITE

EAT MEAL

LARGE
UNBALANCED
MEAL

CRAVINGS

Cravings to Consumption

NEGATIVE
FEEDBACK
LOOP

TIRED,
IRRITABLE, &
DISTRACTED

ENERGY
SLUMPS

LOW ENERGY

pens when the football leaves his hand. If he pays no attention to the result of the throw—the only gauge that allows for improvement—he will be unable to produce a different outcome in the future.

Just as in the case of a quarterback, I contend that the *most* important part of your relationship with food begins immediately *after* eating.

A more empowering way to relate to food is to recognize and *feel* its impact on your body and mind. This relationship, which can literally elevate your existence, is what I call the *Consumption to Freedom* approach. It begins the moment you're finished eating and continues for the next one, two, three, or more hours afterward.

It's the flip side of the cravings, where you switch your focus from how a meal fills the void, or satisfies a craving, to how it *fulfills* your nutritional needs—elevating your mood, energy, and life. To end the dependence on food as a source of immediate gratification and begin to focus on how it enhances your life is the foundation for *Nutritional Freedom*. It lays down the wiring for enjoying the foods that are best for you the most.

Eating what's great for you not *because* it's great for you but because it's what you want to eat, and then because you love the way it makes you feel—that's Nutritional Freedom. It's the sort of freedom that will have you looking at a candy bar and an apple and wanting the apple more than the candy.

Here, you begin to establish and strengthen a positive, life-enhancing relationship with food; consumption for the sake of nourishment. At first it can be a challenge, because it pulls you beyond immediate gratification and calls on you to experience food's ability to uplift and energize.

Rather than using food to stomp out hunger, as one would a campfire—eating vibrant, living food can stoke your fire. It's not the end but the beginning of a period of strength and energy.

THE END OF DIETING

Scaling to the heights of Nutritional Freedom is not the result of discipline, deprivation, or dieting. It is accomplished through the process of strengthening your awareness of food as a source of life fuel—a Transformation as big and important as any you'll ever make.

People with a nearly exclusive Cravings to Consumption relationship will find eliminating unhealthy food and changing eating habits a tremendous challenge. For them, diets are a non-stop test of self-discipline. With little awareness of how food affects their energy and leaves them feeling, there's no feedback, which is essential to self-correction.

Frequently, a person in this predicament attaches to a diet in hopes of being rescued. The result is often a tug-of-war, flexing great discipline to resist the desire to eat. When a dieter recognizes the connection between eating better and feeling better, there's an opening to freedom.

When you become aware that with every bite of food you eat you either pay a price or receive an immediate return, you've taken the first step toward Nutritional Freedom. When you further connect how you feel physically, mentally, and emotionally—not just ten minutes following the meal, but an hour, two, and even three hours later—you've taken the next step. The more you continue to develop and strengthen your awareness of the impact food has on you, the better you will eat, *effortlessly.*

Your current body, health, strength, and fitness are all the result of the decisions you've made so far. If you want to change something about your body and life, the first step is to make better (more life-supportive) choices, which requires a change in your decision-making process. Making intelligent choices—choices that feed your success—means, first and foremost, using your mind, not your stomach, in advance of eating.

Just as you have the freedom to choose to live a life of strength, you have complete and total freedom to choose what you eat. As your awareness grows, your genuine ability to appreciate and enjoy the true pleasure and satisfaction of food will emerge.

The process of cultivating your Nutritional Awareness is the foundation for a lifetime of

Nutritional Freedom—how you eat to live. You can achieve it, step by step, in a reasonable time through the proven, successful, sound strategies in the next chapter. These strategies are the baby steps—the *sets and reps*—of eating that train and strengthen your awareness and will ensure that you *never, ever diet again.*

Here's to a new level of Nutritional Freedom!

CHAPTER 10

Your Path to Nutritional Freedom

Nutritional Awareness is ultimately something you must *experience* and feel to truly under-stand. It's *the* Master Strategy—a practice—on the road to Nutritional Freedom. It's not some-thing that happens overnight, but as you engage the strategies in this chapter you'll start to feel changes almost immediately.

To "be aware" is to be well-informed, alert, and mindful. Nutritionally, it's being aware of both *how* food leaves you feeling and *why* you're eating in the first place. For most people, eat-ing habits are deeply entrenched—far from the light of awareness. That means you don't often recognize destructive eating patterns. And you cannot change what you cannot see. Even when you think you're eating well, in the absence of finely tuned awareness the reality of what you're eating is likely far from ideal.

For example, a popular and healthier option for a quick lunch these days is any one of the fresh-made burrito restaurants. For many, satisfied with having selected a *healthier* option, the critical thinking stops. While they're busy patting themselves on the back for choosing so well, the person behind the counter is heaping on the chicken, rice, beans, cheese, sour cream, and more. Suddenly and unwittingly this healthier, fresher option has become a flour torpedo tip-ping the scales in excess of 1,200 calories, and that's a lot of food for *any* human being.

This is the ideal place to engage awareness in your critical decision making by making a few simple choices: one small scoop of rice and beans, skipping the tortilla, going easy on the cheese, and refusing the sour cream. You've just strengthened your Nutritional Awareness on the way to Nutritional Freedom, and for that, you truly do deserve that pat on the back.

Now you might be thinking, "Okay, I get it. I need to be more aware of what I eat, portions, and how it all affects me. That makes sense. Let's move on."

Not so fast. The decision to tame this burrito is *not* powered by discipline or willpower. Knowing that if you eat too much you will pay later by feeling sluggish is Nutritional Awareness in action. By making informed choices you can both enjoy the burrito while managing the size and content, so your meal leaves you energized and nourished. The stronger your Nutritional Awareness, the easier it is for you to make decisions that elevate you. Naturally, you will be drawn toward making choices that ultimately make you look great, feel great, and live great.

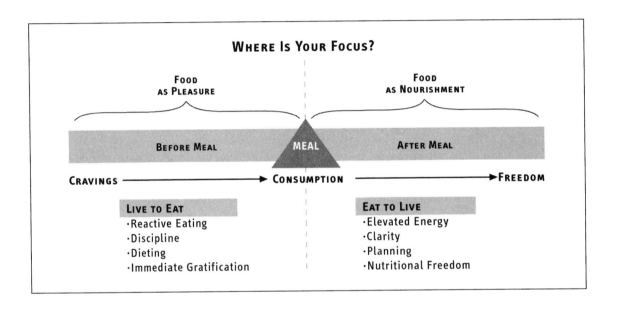

As you train your muscle of Nutritional Awareness during your Transformation, I'll ask you to track the foods you eat and how you feel following each meal. Don't worry—I'm not suggesting that you become some sort of nutritional bookkeeper for the rest of your life. The next 12 weeks is the ideal time to elevate your awareness with this practice.

The goal is to develop *hesitation*, a moment of consideration between the urge to eat and the action. It's in this moment of hesitation that awareness first arises and begins to grow. Until you break the bond between cravings and your conditioned response, you can't even imagine there's a space for hesitation—where freedom could exist. But it's there. I promise.

The more you nourish your body with life-enhancing foods, the more you'll condition yourself to choose the foods that energize your body and elevate your mind. Eventually you will become so accustomed to running on high-grade fuels that nothing less will satisfy.

Be Aware!

To experience how strong your programmed responses can be, try this: The next time your phone rings, let it. Don't reach for it—do not even react! It may sound easy, but when you feel the pull, you'll swear someone else has a hold on your arm. Feeling the desire to pick up that phone is awareness—the gap between action and reaction. The more you practice this pause, the wider it becomes. This is the same pause you can add to your eating, which will be the beginning of Nutritional Freedom. Try it. It's truly enlightening.

The 10 Nutritional Freedom Strategies

10 Start Strong

9 Reclaim Your Kitchen

8 Feed Your Strength After Training

7 Journal Your Way

6 Plan for Success

5 Take the 7th Day Away

4 Make It a Repeat Performance

3 Eat Early and Often

2 Make Protein the Centerpiece

1 Keep It Balanced

NUTRITIONAL FREEDOM

NUTRITIONAL AWARENESS

UNCONSCIOUS REACTIVE EATING

Each of the ten strategies following is designed to enhance and support your Nutritional Awareness and a lifetime of Nutritional Freedom. Read them all now, then come back to them over the course of your Transformation to fully embrace them a step at a time.

NUTRITIONAL FREEDOM STRATEGY NO. 1: KEEP IT BALANCED

I'm sure you're aware of at least one of the many popular diets that involve taking one macronutrient way out of balance. Take your pick: low-fat, low-carb, no-carb. Perhaps you've tried one of these diets yourself. If so, you too may have discovered these are not long-term strategies. While producing some temporary results, these diets tend to fall short on their promises over the long haul.

Thankfully, there is one sane strategy for eating that has proven effective in swapping body fat for lean muscle, keeping you vibrant and strong. It's not a diet but a guiding practice for setting you on your journey to Nutritional Freedom. This nonsecret is to eat sensible, nutrient-rich meals, with the right balance of proteins, carbohydrates, and essential fats.

When you eat this way, the intelligent appetite you misinterpreted as a craving—"get me a double-double cheeseburger now"—is completely erased. Every time you choose to fuel your body with balanced nutrition you take a step toward freedom, a life of strength, energy, and vitality.

Macronutrient Balance

When I mention *macronutrients,* I'm referring to proteins, carbohydrates, and fats. These three primary nutrients are essential in the largest amount for your body. In contrast, *micronutrients*—naturally found in many of your macronutrient sources—are the numerous vitamins, minerals, antioxidants, and other life-enhancing nutrients needed in smaller quantities. Here's a brief overview of macronutrients:

Protein, from the Greek word *protas,* meaning "of primary importance," is essential to the structure and function of every cell in your body. In addition to its leading role in the formation of muscle, protein can elevate your mood, increase mental focus, sustain energy, and support your metabolism. Most of your brain's chemical messengers—neurotransmitters—are made from amino acids, the building blocks of protein. The effectiveness of protein in supporting fat loss and lasting satiety (freedom from cravings and hunger) has made it the star of weight-loss programs. As the knowledge of the power of protein continues to grow, so does my contention that it is those who do *not* exercise regularly that *most need* protein.

Carbohydrates are the macronutrient you don't want to meet in a dark alley alone. They've really taken a beating in recent years—which is both too bad and a good thing. It's a good thing in that people need to become more aware and respectful of them. Our unregistered carbohydrate intake—those snacks that seem to not even count—has been (and continues for many) to be off the charts. The bad part is that it's not the carbs that are evil—in fact, carbohydrates are the primary and essential source of energy for your entire body and mind. They fuel your nervous system, brain, and muscles. Carbs keep you moving, working, training, and living.

The biggest issue is how refined carbohydrates, when consumed in excess, apart from a complete meal, spike insulin off the charts. For example, nondiet soda can easily contain 13 teaspoons of refined sugar—the resulting spike in insulin will trigger fat storage and prohibit the use of fat as fuel.

As part of a well-balanced meal, carbohydrates help the effective delivery of proteins and tell the brain, "You've got energy." For that reason, almost every meal should include both protein and carbs.

Stick with complex carbohydrates, those found in nature, such as brown rice and sweet potatoes (see the Approved Foods list). Complex carbs gradually release into your body, providing sustained energy, optimal delivery of nutrients, and longer-lasting satiety than simple carbs do.

Veggies and most fruits you'd see at the farmer's market are good sources of energy and rich in vital nutrients (vitamins, minerals, antioxidants, and fiber). While I highly recommend several servings of fruit a day, some are more likely to spike insulin than others. So choose your fruits wisely.

Fats in the 1990s were the villain of nutrition. Today, most of us know that fats, like people, aren't all bad—and some are even essential to life. Now the focus is on increasing our intake of the health-promoting essential fats—while curtailing our intake of the unhealthy fats (including the saturated and *trans* fats).

Essential fats, including omega-3s, omega-6s, and others, are *vital* for your optimal physical and mental performance. They provide fuel for energy, support fat loss, and promote optimal cellular health.

How to Build a Meal

When you set out to build a balanced meal, consider these simple guidelines: Don't get all caught up in counting calories. Instead, I suggest you focus on portions. A portion, one serving, should be about the same size as the palm of your hand.

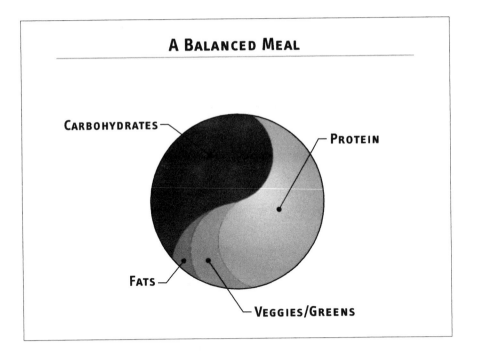

A BALANCED MEAL

CARBOHYDRATES

PROTEIN

FATS

VEGGIES/GREENS

Your first step is to select a quality source of lean protein. Then balance it with an equal portion of a complex carbohydrate. As for fat, it's more an issue of getting bad fats out and then finding some good (essential) fat in your day—not each meal. Select foods that have low saturated fat. That means during your Transformation the fattiest cuts of red meat are out—except on your once-a-week free day (Strategy No. 5). Be vigilant about minimizing the obvious saturated fats (cheeses, butter, and the like).

Ah, and as for veggies, which few of us are guilty of overeating, I like to aim high and shoot for a main course vegetable portion and include a leafy green, like a fresh salad.

This way of crafting a meal, repeated day in and day out, will help you produce the results you truly desire. It's a lifestyle you can thrive on, not a diet to "survive" on. I've practiced this same sound, balanced approach to optimal nutrition for years. The fact that this is not the sort of radical diet tomfoolery that garners front page news might just be reason enough to give it a try.

When Building a Balanced Meal:

- Portions should be palm-size.
- Start with a serving of lean protein.
- Balance with an equal portion of an acceptable carbohydrate.
- Include essential fats daily.
- Add at least one serving of vegetables twice daily.

NUTRITIONAL FREEDOM STRATEGY NO. 2: MAKE PROTEIN THE CENTERPIECE

If you've been following the latest scientific weight loss trends or have been enjoying a fit lifestyle for any length of time, you know the importance of eating quality protein. It provides the "building blocks" for your muscles, skin, tendons, and every cell in your body. Protein also supports your immune system, promotes stable energy levels, and stimulates your metabolism, which is helpful for encouraging fat loss. For all of these reasons, protein should be the centerpiece for every meal.

In addition to its role in the regeneration and building of lean muscle, protein is the most thermogenic macronutrient, which means it's less likely than carbs or fats to be stored as body fat. Your body has to work hard to break down protein, which means there's a boost to your metabolism. As an added bonus, up to 30 percent of its caloric value is lost during this process.

Protein, as part of a balanced meal, slows the release of carbohydrates, producing a favorable insulin response. This means hours of freedom from hunger. If you've ever experienced the "Chinese food phenomenon," where you're starving 15 minutes after dinner, then you know how quickly simple carbs, like white rice, can leave you craving more.

Carbohydrates are plentiful. Go to any restaurant and watch as they're piled on before, during, and after dinner. Carbs are cheap and often lead to portion distortion. The way most places serve up the bread and mashed potatoes in comparison to the chicken, you'd think protein was more precious than gold.

The absence of protein, and its capacity to buffer the release of carbohydrates, is another reason why the great American pastime of snacking on high-carbohydrate foods—be it baked chips or fat-free cookies—is so detrimental. The overhyped fat-free snack foods are nothing more than high-glycemic carbs that quickly skyrocket your insulin and put fat storage into high gear. Snacking is an unconscious, addictive habit that is a quick road to "mysterious" weight gain.

Order Up!

You must take control and flex your muscles of Nutritional Awareness. Whenever or wherever you eat—at home, on the road, or on the go—make the selection of a source of quality protein job number one. If you do that, everything else will fall into place.

For breakfast it might be egg whites, for lunch and dinner fish, chicken, or turkey. Another popular way to get your protein is with a high-quality nutrition shake—a discovery more people are making every day.

When dining out, be selective and ask for what you want. If you want the chicken without the sauce, then ask. If you want only egg whites, ask. You might be surprised how many restaurants, large and small, happily accommodate your requests.

Four Tips to Make Protein the Centerpiece:

- Eat protein with *every* meal.
- When planning, ordering, or cooking your meal, start with your lean protein source and build from there.
- When consuming your meal, enjoy at least part of your lean protein first.
- Keep your meals balanced.

NUTRITIONAL FREEDOM STRATEGY NO. 3: EAT EARLY AND OFTEN

Five Circles Beats Three Squares Any Day

"Three squares a day." So ingrained is it in our culture and minds that it's less a social agreement than a natural occurrence like the setting of the sun. The sun comes up, we eat three meals, the sun sets, we sleep.

Today, even with the three-square-meals-a-day ritual imprinted in our cultural DNA, Americans have by and large distorted this golden rule beyond recognition. We skip breakfast, eat quick lunches, slug down coffee, snack throughout the day to compensate for the poor start, and then consume more than half of our daily calories in one meal: dinner. This is a perfect meal plan *if* you're looking to slow your metabolism to a crawl, stunt your cognitive performance, and pack on body fat at record speed. And as you recall from Chapter 1 the formula is working to near perfection.

At the risk of coming off as a bit of a heretic, three squares a day is not the only way to eat. The three-meals-a-day plan is the product of a different time and a much different world. Food was less available, less processed, and people were more active. It was a fine idea and served us well, but it's time to face the fact that three squares a day is the fossil fuel of eating. There is a better way.

Eating five to six compact meals approximately every three hours throughout the day is the absolute best and most efficient way to stoke your metabolism, keep your energy high, body strong, and mind alert—it helps you feel great. When you eat this way you make better, clearer, stronger choices about how and what you eat.

Rather than going six or more hours without eating, consuming smaller meals more often is an effective way to avoid overeating. Take too much time between meals, and you're more likely to become ravenously hungry before the next. As a result, you often choose to eat meals that are too large. And if you eat more than you actually need, you will store the extra calories as fat and add stress to your body.

Eating more often is not only better for your waistline, but keeps your blood sugar stable, your metabolism humming steadily, and helps you avoid running to the vending machine for that quick "pick-me-up" candy, soft drink, or energy drink.

Five-a-Day for Life

In *Body-for-LIFE* my brother was one of the first to take the idea of smaller, more frequent meals beyond a theory and put it into action. His Transformation program called for six smaller meals about every three hours; three whole food meals and three in the form of convenient, easy-to-prepare nutrition shakes to ensure optimal levels of nutrients.

It's a rock-solid plan. On paper. In a *perfect* world, you would eat a *perfectly* balanced meal with the *perfect* balance of protein, carbohydrates, and vegetables every three hours. But it's *not* a perfect world. And, here's where I must come in with a confession: I've never quite been able to make six meals per day consistently. Even at my best I've come back time and again to my standard *five meals per day.*

A Plan to Remember

I admit that six meals deserves a four-star rating, but you can succeed in your Transformation with five sound, balanced meals per day—*and* without every meal being perfectly divisible by five. That means your "five circles" do not have to be the exact same size.

Place your full attention on achieving three smaller, well-balanced, nutritious meals first— your three pillars. Get them right and eat well. The other two (midmorning and midafternoon) in-between-meals meals can be more along the lines of a balanced, nutritious full-strength snack or a quality nutrition shake. I do not suggest you drop your standards to allow for "energy" bars or the low-grade liquid protein potions in the ready-to-drink aisles.

I'm very careful about how I use the term "snack" to describe the in-between-meals meals. The reason is simple. I believe the word snack is synonymous with vending machines, junk food, or something you feed the dog. At the very least, a snack sounds like something inferior to a meal. Thus, I use the term snack to describe a healthy, nutritious smaller portion of food.

This modified "3 + 2 plan" enables nearly everyone to make the five-meal grade and enjoy its many benefits. Plus, you'll be relieved to know you don't have to pull out the chicken breast, rice, and veggies at ten-thirty in the morning for all to stare at.

I'll end this strategy with the following simple and memorable formula for living long and strong. Once you hear it, you won't forget. Once you adopt it, it will change your life. It consists of a few magic words of wisdom that my friend, Tom Bilella (whom I introduced you to in Chapter 5) shares with his clients: "It's easy, all you have to do is three by three, and five by nine."

Translated, Tom advocates eating three meals by 3:00 P.M. and five meals by 9:00 P.M. Staying properly fueled throughout the day keeps you operating at optimal levels. The late afternoon meal helps you avert crashes, and your last meal closes out your day as you began: strong. Finish the last meal before 9:00 P.M.; save your nights for restful sleep and recovery.

Of course, your last meal might be by 7:30 P.M., as in the following example.

My sample meal schedule looks like this: 7:00 A.M. breakfast, 10:00 A.M. in-between-meal meal, 1:00 P.M. lunch, 4:00 P.M. in-between-meal meal, and a 7:30 P.M. dinner.

Simple Rules to Live By:

- **Eat five reasonably balanced meals each day.**
- **Adopt a 3 + 2 plan to ensure your five-meal success.**
- **Consider using a quality nutrition shake in your daily plan.**
- **Remember the 3 × 3, 5 × 9 rule.**

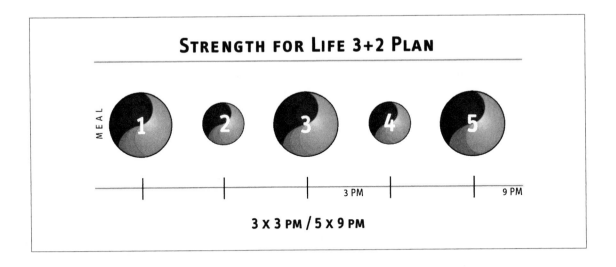

STRENGTH FOR LIFE 3+2 PLAN

MEAL

1   2   3   4   5

3 PM   9 PM

3 X 3 PM / 5 X 9 PM

Shaken Not Stirred

If you're barely eating three decent meals a day now, the idea of preparing five perfectly balanced meals can be nothing short of daunting. For anyone. The thought of *adding* not one but two meals per day can leave you shaking your head.

So how do you overcome the seemingly time-consuming, logistically terrifying dilemma of eating five meals?

Ladies and gentlemen, I give you: the nutrition shake. More convenient than a fast-food drive-through, a nutrition shake can quickly provide your body and mind with a complete array of vital nutrients to nourish and energize you.

For over 15 years my ritual of enjoying two nutrition shakes a day, nearly every day, has been a vital source of energy, strength, and nutrition. In early 1990, I helped launch the world's first meal-replacement shake, an entirely new concept that would become the largest single category in nutrition within the decade.

Often misunderstood, many people still believe that a nutrition shake is a protein supplement for bodybuilders, a high-fat liquid calorie supplement for the elderly, or a drink supplement for dieters. While many nutrition shakes have been cast as supplements, I contend that none of the above is even remotely accurate.

If you desire a strong, lean body, feeling energized and nourished, a high-quality nutrition shake can save your day and make your life. You'll want a shake that provides a blend of protein, complex carbohydrates, essential fats, dietary fiber, vitamins, and minerals. It can be the perfect "midair refueling" meal for elevating your body and mind—delivering a full spectrum of balanced nutrition in minutes.

Once you've experienced how much easier a nutrition shake can make the five circles way of eating, and witness its *transformative* powers, you'll never go back to the prehistoric three squares. That much I can promise you.

I believe that in the next decade we will transform the shape of our country. In support of this vision I have created *Full Strength,* the next-generation nutrition shake—the future of fast food. In the next ten years, as more and more people come to embrace this evolution in convenient, delicious nutrition, I see the nutrition shake becoming the predominant form of fast food in America. I'm not suggesting food will become nutrition shakes, but rather that nutrition shakes will be more widely accepted as food.

Today I enjoy two Full Strength shakes every day because of the way it makes me feel. It's sure-fire

continued on next page

nutrition that uplifts my mind, is pure pleasure for my senses, and gets me back on task in minutes, not hours. Not just back in flow, but at a *new level* of energy for up to four solid hours of energy and focus. It's my secret weapon for creating more time in my day and meeting the increasing demands of life. And with a taste so decadent you won't believe it's great for you, it's my five-minute "shake break" revival that I look forward to with a sense of anticipation. There's something very reassuring in knowing that at least one meal a day is balanced, nutrient-rich, and portion controlled.

Enjoying nutrition shakes is not mandatory for your Transformation—but it undeniably provides a strategic advantage. One nutrition shake (and in some cases two) can be a great boost.

Clinical Study Shows Full Strength Nutrition Shakes Superior to Exercise Alone

In a 2007 clinical study conducted at the University of Oklahoma, subjects (adult men and women) followed a basic exercise program for 10 weeks. The participants were placed in two groups: exercise-only or exercise plus two *Full Strength*® premium nutrition shakes each day. No other dietary restrictions were placed on either group.

After just ten weeks the exercise group who consumed the *Full Strength* premium nutrition shakes daily had experienced significant improvements over the regular food group, including:

- 83 percent greater reduction in total body fat
- 59 percent greater increase in muscle mass
- 65 percent drop in total cholesterol
- 50 percent greater increase in endurance performance
- 44 percent greater reduction in fatigue (increased energy)

Most remarkably, the *Full Strength* group was able to simultaneously lose body fat and gain lean muscle without *any dietary restrictions* or caloric deprivation.

This study, concluded in December 2007, is unlike any other nutrition shake study ever conducted, as this was the first study to provide a nutrition shake to overweight and borderline obese adults in which there was no typical diet intervention.

According to director Jeffrey R. Stout, Ph.D., at the Department of Health and Exercise Science at the University of Oklahoma, *"Based on nutritional analysis, I believe the significantly better results were due to Full Strength improving the participants' overall diet."*

NUTRITIONAL FREEDOM STRATEGY NO. 4:
MAKE IT A REPEAT PERFORMANCE

We have such a wonderful and overwhelming variety of food from which to choose, and it seems we take advantage of it. Chinese food today, Mexican tomorrow, and Thai the next day—31 flavors in 22 ever-larger sizes. This unlimited variety does just what it is intended to do: It fuels our desire for more. We eat more when presented with an assortment of foods—according to research as much as 50 percent more calories than when we have only one choice.

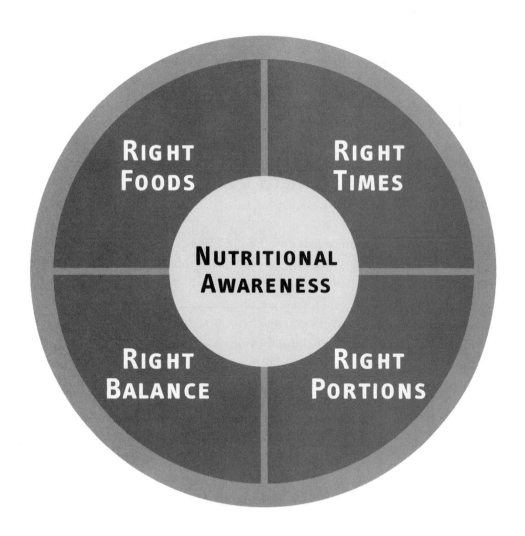

My staple meals are not a creative exercise in culinary arts. For the most part I eat the same foods day in and day out. My breakfast and in-between-meal meals are typically repeat performances, while my lunch and dinners are where variety comes to life. I find this saves time and simplifies my life greatly. Even shopping becomes easier. When I go to the grocery store, it's the same aisles, same selections.

If you enjoy food like I do, keeping it simple does not mean you have to sacrifice variety. You can go all out enjoying extravagant meals on special occasions, but day to day, it's best to follow repeat patterns of eating consistent foods for nourishment. This can make your life easier and propel your success. Make simplicity your strength for the 12 weeks of Transformation. Establish a set pattern, make some staple meals, limit variety, and repeat.

Keep It Simple:

- Choose balanced meals that nourish you and stick to them.
- Appreciate your meals for both the taste and how the food makes you feel.
- Make every day a repeat performance, not every meal.
- Enjoy a wide variety of foods daily.

NUTRITIONAL FREEDOM STRATEGY NO. 5: TAKE THE 7TH DAY AWAY

Take one day a week and relax; enjoy a day off. Perhaps there's one "bad" food you feel you just can't live without. If you want Chicago deep-dish pizza followed by some cheesecake and vanilla Swiss almond ice cream later on in the day, go for it. This is your day off. But beware: An all-day food bender may leave you feeling terrible, because you will now be making the connection between what you eat and how you feel.

Knowing you have one day off is helpful for your mental well-being. Please, don't fall into the trap of thinking that if you restrict yourself from free days you'll make progress faster; this often isn't the case. It's important for you to let yourself relax, put down your strategies, and eat whatever you like on your day off. This not only provides additional calories your body may need to recover from intense training, but also recharges and rejuvenates, so you come back to your overall nutritional plan with greater commitment.

Following the age-old wisdom that we learn the most from our mistakes, keep your daily nutrition journal during your 7th day. The foods you may choose to eat can have a profound impact on how you feel. This is one of the best times to closely track the effect different foods have on you.

For the 7th Day:

- Choose a consistent day of the week to enjoy your day off—a floating day does not work.
- Synchronize your nutritional day off with your training day off.
- Keep your daily nutrition journal.

After the 7th Day:
How to Have Your Cake and Eat It Too

The promise of Nutritional Freedom is delivered through strengthening your muscle of Nutritional Awareness. You must be able to create a pause and begin seeing through cravings the instant they arise. Remember, your freedom is in the space between temptation and reaction.

Here's a saying I often use that captures the essence of Nutritional Freedom: "You can't have your cake and eat it too, until you can have your cake and *not* eat it."

It's as much a life principle as it is about sensible eating. Whether it's cake, shopping, or love—only when you're fully content without them will any of these be an appreciated addition to your life. Otherwise, you're eating and consuming out of weakness rather than the strength of gratitude.

Here's what you're going to do: During the first week of your Transformation, buy, make, or bake the food you most crave when you want to indulge or treat yourself. Get it by Thursday because you're going to indulge on Sunday—or your 7th day. You should be aware of this favorite indulgence so you can experience not eating it, even knowing you will in a few short days.

For this example we'll use one of my favorites: a creamy, rich, dark chocolate layer cake. When you see the cake in the fridge, listen closely to your inner dialogue. Feel the temptation and desire to act that leaps up. You might even decide to record it in your journal. Putting words to your desire for food is a great way to create some distance. It helps give you perspective and expands the space between craving and reaction.

Keep with your experience—monitoring it Friday and Saturday. No slips. Then come Sunday, set aside 15 minutes to indulge. But don't just dig in as you normally would. Instead, enjoy each and every bite as though it was your *very* first taste of this favorite food.

That's right. Rather than enjoying the first bite or two and slipping into full-consumption mode, which is the normal way, you're going to take 15 first bites (yes, 15 first bites) of this amazing, delicious chocolate cake. Make certain you taste and enjoy the last bite as much as you did the first.

As for what, if anything, may surprise you, I'll leave that for you to discover.

Bon appetit!

NUTRITIONAL FREEDOM STRATEGY NO. 6: PLAN FOR SUCCESS

Eating is one of life's great pleasures, and at times a tremendous inconvenience. It takes time out of our busy days—time that we'd like to give to other, seemingly more important things. Ironically, the more we attempt to "save time" by avoiding eating or neglecting nutrition, the more power food exerts in our life. Eventually we're left powerless. Hunger seeks its revenge and begins taking control without regard for health, energy, or impact on strength.

"Failure to plan is a plan for failure" is as true for your nutrition as it is for your life. When you allow yourself to be in a reactive relationship with eating, you're setting yourself up for one failure after another and a long road ahead. No amount of willpower can sustain itself in this sort of environment.

Eating right can take an incredible amount of effort and discipline or some up-front planning. When you eat on a regular schedule and plan ahead—anticipating the need for nourishment—you will eat better food. Why? Because keeping yourself properly fueled enables you to activate your higher mind, the decision-making center of the brain called the *prefrontal cortex.*

With your critical thinking engaged, you remain in control and free to choose what you eat, wisely. Conversely, ignore the need for nourishment and your *thinking* will arise from the "lower," more primitive brain. This most likely causes you to eat in reaction to cravings, and you will likely be out of control. The result is often uncontrollable splurges on empty-calorie destructive foods.

Don't allow yourself to become a victim of reactive eating. Adopt a daily practice of writing down your plan for tomorrow, even if you know that three of your meals are going to be the same as today. Do it every day, six days per week. This will bring both consistency and rhythm to your eating.

Plan Your Meal Plan

According to many of those who complete a Transformation, the dedication to planning nutrition in advance is one of the key contributors to success. If you've been out of practice or have never planned your meals in advance, now's the time to take it on again or for the first time.

Prior to the close of each day, look forward and plan your meals. Don't wait for the momentary whim of desire to direct what you will eat. Plan for clarity and to eliminate the need to put together meals on the spot.

Use the daily nutrition tracker pages or keep a spiral notebook and be sure to plan your

SAMPLE DAILY MEAL PLANS

Time	Meal
6:00 am	Full Strength® Premium Nutrition Shake, Chocolate
9:00 am	Low-fat cottage cheese & fresh raspberries, water
12:00 pm	Grilled chicken breast, brown rice, fresh vegetables, water
3:00 pm	Full Strength® Premium Nutrition Shake, Vanilla
6:00 pm	Broiled salmon, steamed brown rice, steamed spinach, water

Time	Meal
7:00 am	6 egg-white omelet w/ low-fat cheese, oatmeal with honey, water
10:00 am	Full Strength® Premium Nutrition Shake, Vanilla
1:00 pm	Turkey sandwich with lettuce, onions, and tomatoes on whole-wheat bread; small serving of coleslaw; water w/ lemon
4:00 pm	Full Strength® Premium Nutrition Shake, Chocolate
7:00 pm	Grilled chicken breast, fettuccine & low-fat pasta sauce, baby spinach, water

Time	Meal
8:00 am	6 scrambled egg whites with red and green bell peppers, onions, and low-fat cheddar cheese; 1 slice of whole-wheat toast; water
11:00 am	Full Strength® Premium Nutrition Shake, Chocolate
2:00 pm	Grilled chicken breast, baked sweet potato, fresh vegetables, water w/ lemon
5:00 pm	Blended low-fat cottage cheese and fresh organic blueberries, water
8:00 pm	Romaine chicken salad with cucumber, red onion, red bell pepper; tomatoes, with light honey-Dijon salad dressing

mealtimes (7-10-1-4-7, for example). Write in your journal the food you plan on consuming for each meal. Do this each night.

Finally, have a plan for those times when you do fall into a reactive mode with food. Have a strategy to get back on course if you miss a meal, find yourself out to lunch with a friend from out of town, or something else has gotten you off course.

Three Tips to Keep You on Course:

- Plan tomorrow's meals today.
- Follow your plan.
- Have a contingency plan.

NUTRITIONAL FREEDOM STRATEGY NO. 7: JOURNAL YOUR WAY

Grab a sheet of paper and quickly write down everything you ate yesterday.

Are you done? This is not an attempt to test your memory but rather to make the point that for most of us it's easier to recall what we did socially, with friends or family, or what we achieved at work, than what we ate. The ability to recall is indicative of having given it thought in advance. It demonstrates eating with awareness. When you do something out of habit, there's little recall.

For the duration of your 12-week Transformation Training Camp you will be keeping a nutrition journal, tracking what you eat and the peaks and valleys in your energy, concentration, and mood throughout each day. In my years of experience, I've found this to be the single most powerful practice for boosting Nutritional Awareness.

The rules are simple: If you bite it, write it. *Everything* you eat or drink is promptly captured in your journal. Be sure to write down what goes into your mouth in one column and track your energy levels and mood in the other (this could be 5 minutes, 20 minutes, or an hour later). After just a week of journaling, expect to be shocked by the reality of what you're eating. Even people who assume they're in tune with what they eat, who swear their diets are "excellent," are often faced with a completely different reality.

While you'll likely find that your prime-time meals could use some tune-up, the real shock may come when you see the amount of calorie leakage—the in-between meal snacking and random bites that are generally just ignored. Believe me, until you write down the specifics of each meal along with everything in between, you don't truly know what is going into your body. Once you take into account that *every* bite of food either nourishes success or feeds failure, you can see how important it is to be more careful about what you eat.

NAME _Shawn_

DATE _6/23_   WEEK _7_

	FOODS and BEVERAGES CONSUMED	BODY + MIND STATE	WATER/TIME
MEAL #1 Time: 7:35 AM ☒ PM [ ]	Full Strength Vanilla Shake w/ 6 organic raspberries - made with 15 oz water	Immediate surge of energy after my morning workout. Feel confident, focused & clear. Ready for a great day!	16 oz/6:30 15 oz/ with shake
MEAL #2 Time: 10:30 AM ☒ PM [ ]	1 Fuji apple, 2 cups non-fat cottage cheese, 2 oz. raw almonds	Still going strong. Not overly full and love the apples with the almonds.	16 oz/9:45 16 oz/noon
MEAL #3 Time: 1:00 AM [ ] PM ☒	1 full grilled chicken breast 1 cup brown rice 1 cup steamed veggies @Tokyo Joe's w/teriyaki sauce	Stopped short on the rice as the bowl was big. Tastes great and can feel slight slowing as my body receives the food.	8 oz/1:30
MEAL #4 Time: 3:45 AM [ ] PM ☒	1 perfect chocolate Full Strength. Just added 16 oz water and ice and I'm going strong in minutes.	Yummmmm...perfect mid-day refuel. My energy is elevated, I'm free to fully engage until dinner.	16 oz/ with shake
MEAL #5 Time: 6:35 AM [ ] PM ☒	Fresh Wild Salmon, 1-yam w/ 1 tbsp. "non-butter" butter, 1-cup steamed spinach, 1-fresh salad w/ balsamic dressing	Perfect dinner. Thanks to afternoon refuel I'm hungry but not ravenous. Portions were right and I feel great.	16 oz/5:15 16 oz/8:15
OTHER Time: 10:00 AM [ ] PM ☒	1 "Fage" brand fat-free yogurt with sliced strawberries	This is the perfect Greek yogurt. Great protein, low carbs and no fat. Great snack for my evening.	8 oz/10:00

You can create a Food Journal out of any spiral notebook, or copy the Nutritional Tracker page from this book (Appendix C). There are also forms you can download from MyStrength forLife.com. Either way, keep your journal handy at all times—make it easy to write things down immediately and consistently.

Helpful Journal Guidelines:

- If you bite it, write it (this includes all beverages).
- Include portion sizes and how you feel following each meal.
- Note your energy levels and moods periodically throughout the day.
- Tracking your food intake is not the same as planning your meals.

NUTRITIONAL FREEDOM STRATEGY NO. 8:
FEED YOUR STRENGTH AFTER TRAINING

It's a common misconception that strength training leads to fuller, stronger muscles. While it's true training is the stimulus for growth, it's the recovery and proper nourishment immediately following your training that fuel your muscles, energy, and strength.

Intense training leaves your muscles screaming for vital nutrients necessary for rebuilding your body stronger. Yet, you don't experience this post-workout hunger, for it's on a cellular level. In fact, you may not feel hungry at all after working out. Even worse, you may intentionally avoid eating as a weight loss strategy, thinking, "Why eat, I just worked out and burned off all those calories?"

Regardless of how you feel immediately following your training, this is the right time to infuse your muscles with high-quality proteins, carbohydrates, and other essential nutrients. As soon as your workout is over the clock starts ticking—the sooner you shuttle in optimal nutrition, the better. Most experts agree that the first 30 to 45 minutes following your training are the most critical to capture the full benefits of your hard work.

Following exercise, your body exhibits an elevated metabolic rate, much as it does upon awakening. Starving yourself following training throws you into a catabolic state, breaking down muscle tissue. As a result, your hard effort goes unrewarded and you've actually elevated your body's ability to store fat.

Set Your Place at the Training Table:

- Make sure you eat within 45 minutes after training.
- This is an ideal place for a convenient quality nutrition shake.
- Consume high-quality protein for full recovery.
- Enjoy additional carbohydrates after your workout to replenish energy.

NUTRITIONAL FREEDOM STRATEGY NO. 9:
RECLAIM YOUR KITCHEN

It's difficult to do the right thing in the wrong environment. To avoid making your each and every day a test of discipline and willpower, be prepared, just like the Boy Scouts. Set yourself up for success.

The New Microwave

If you have memories of the 1970s that don't come from TV, you may recall when the microwave oven became a fixture in U.S. homes. This "space-age" device was going to revolutionize the way we eat, making delicious meals more convenient than ever.

Over three decades later, the most excitement the microwave has delivered is a few sparks when accidentally placing foil in it. As for cooking food, it's become a glorified, oversized toaster. It's basically used to heat things like the trays of frozen, processed food we throw into it. And, speaking of the ever-handy toaster, I'll bet you have one proudly adorning your countertops. What does it do? Crisp up bread so you can butter and jam the already high-glycemic treat and toast frozen waffles (or worse).

I'm not suggesting you trash your reheating devices, but rather consider that the most versatile appliance—the one that can have the greatest impact on your strength and vitality—could be stored in your cupboards right now. I'm talking about the most frequently used appliance in our kitchen: the blender.

Today's modern, high-capacity blenders are amazingly versatile appliances capable of delivering high-quality nutrition quickly. One of the reasons I've become so blender savvy is that I use them to make delicious nutrition shakes every day. As you move up from the run-of-the-mill blenders, the things you can do with them become ever more impressive.

Of course, being the blender aficionado that I am, I don't have just *any* blender. I've upgraded to the Ferrari of blenders, also known as the Blendtec Total Blender. It's the very same single-push-button, auto-programmed, mixing *hot-rod* blender you see behind the counters at Starbucks and many smoothie joints. I kid you not, this machine is powerful enough to nearly boil water or make snow! It delivers fast, convenient, and wholesome food in moments. Toss in a load of fresh vegetables, push the button, and you can make soup in less than two minutes. You can even make your own peanut butter, fresh smoothies, and much more.

If you're one of those people whose parents passed down the myth that blenders should be hidden away after use like small firearms, you can put that myth to rest. If there is anything that shows off your Nutritional Awareness, it's having your blender, bright and shiny, sitting smack dab in the center of your countertop and placing your toaster in a cupboard, where it belongs.

In the case of your Transformation, this means reclaiming your kitchen: It's out with the old, in with the new. This starts with removing temptation—make your home a "junk-free" zone. With only strong food options in your kitchen, you'll find it easier to make the right choices.

Keep your refrigerator and pantry stocked with the foods that keep you running at your peak. Remember, people who make the right choices do not have extra willpower or discipline. They've set themselves up for success.

About every four weeks, reclaim your kitchen. Here's how it works: In the morning after breakfast (so you're not hungry) begin by scouting your kitchen. Look through your refrigerator, freezer, and pantry. When you find a "bad" food, one that has mysteriously appeared, toss it out and write it on a list. When you're done going through every nook and cranny, look at the list of things removed and then replace each with a food from the "good" list (in Appendix B).

How to Reclaim Your Kitchen:

- First, remove your hunger by enjoying a balanced meal.
- Open this book to the approved food list.
- Clean out all foods that are not going to move you in the right direction.
- Replace the "bad" foods with the right foods to fuel your success.

NUTRITION FREEDOM STRATEGY NO. 10: START STRONG

What if you went 12, 14, or even 16 hours without eating? You'd be starving, cranky, exhausted, and unable to think straight, all while your metabolism slowed to conserve energy. To make matters worse, your body would be stockpiling as much fat as possible. More ready for hibernation than battle, the last thing you'd want is to confront any performance demands. Yet this is precisely what more than half of Americans do every single day when they lumber into the world sluggish from head to toe, having missed the most important meal of the day: breakfast.

Skipping breakfast is a devastating nutritional mistake.

Without breakfast, your body dives into starvation mode. Your metabolism slows down to a crawl, and you're inclined to overeat on unhealthy foods later. Many people contend that they don't have time to eat. Others confuse skipping breakfast with a weight-loss strategy when the reality is the opposite; they're actually stunting their strength, slowing their brains, elevating stress, and increasing fat storage.

Eating breakfast on a regular basis is one of the key behaviors among individuals who are

DO YOU START STRONG?

PEOPLE WHO EAT BREAKFAST:	PEOPLE WHO SKIP BREAKFAST:
• Start their day strong	• Are in starvation mode, increasing stress
• Show greater focus and energy	• Have low energy and loss of focus
• Boost their metabolism all day	• Slow their metabolism to save energy
• Eat healthier and smaller dinners	• Eat larger unbalanced meals
• Are less likely to overeat	• Tend to binge on junk food

successful at losing weight and maintaining that weight loss. According to the National Weight Control Registry, of people who have successfully lost an average of 70 pounds and kept it off for six years, only 4 percent said they ever skipped breakfast. Experts say that's because breakfast eaters are more likely to have a structured eating plan throughout the day and consequently are less likely to overeat or snack between meals.

Eating Just "Any" Breakfast Isn't Good Enough

Unfortunately, of the many who *do* eat breakfast, what they are eating may be worse than skipping it altogether. Starting the day with a bagel, doughnut, sweet cereal, or other refined carbohydrates can create a sudden burst of insulin, causing blood sugar to drop. An hour or two later they may start feeling edgy, irritable, and unable to concentrate and are driven to eat more simple carbs to compensate.

In contrast, a balanced breakfast with lean protein, complex carbohydrates, and fiber actually revs you up for the day. Your body is at its metabolic peak in the morning, so calories consumed early in the day are least likely to put on pounds.

Breakfast Eaters Think Better and Are Thinner

Those who do eat a sound breakfast not only function better physically and mentally but are also thinner than those who skip it. You may have noticed this in your own life. Skipping breakfast sets you up for compulsive snacking later, which leads to weight gain. Start your day on empty and your willpower will be no match for the cravings that follow.

A Harvard Medical School survey found that children who ate breakfast had notable gains in academic and emotional function, better grades, attendance, behavior, and psychological test scores. Lest you think this is any different for adults, skipping breakfast has been shown to have a negative impact on mental performance all day. A study published in *The American Journal of Clinical Nutrition* showed that eating breakfast improves adult performance on memory tests.

Research supports the sound advice *Sesame Street* has offered kids for nearly 40 years: A well-balanced breakfast is the only way to start a great day. When you start strong, you've set yourself on the course for success all day.

Here's How to Start Strong:

- **Enjoy a balanced breakfast every day.**
- **Avoid simple refined carbs.**

NUTRITION TIPS

Simple Tips, Tricks, and Techniques for Eating Right

Tip: Get More Fiber, Regularly

Fiber is vital to your heart and colon health. It improves gastrointestinal functioning, helps prevent colon cancer, and reduces cholesterol. Fiber also increases satiety after meals by helping you feel full longer.

You can get fiber from fruits, leafy greens, and whole grain products. People who follow strict low-carb diets must be very attentive, and are well advised to supplement their fiber intake. Aim for 30 grams or more of fiber a day.

Tip: Drink H$_2$O for Life

Hydration is more important than most think. Even slight dehydration can cause your physical *and* mental performance to plummet. Dehydration increases the toxins in your body, slows your metabolism, accelerates aging, and even elevates the risk of a number of illnesses, including cancer.

Drink eight to ten glasses or more of water every day. If you're training, which I like to imagine you are, you may consider this a minimum. Your body best utilizes water if you make a habit of drinking it regularly rather than chugging a glass every hour or so.

Tip: Use Sports Drinks for . . . Sports

Please understand that these brightly colored, exotic flavored performance drinks are often extremely high in sugar—and in some cases loaded with the worst of sugars. Sure, there are electrolytes for that postmarathon depletion, but they are not a replacement for water. If you absolutely must have your "ade"—great! Slam one down after you've climbed off the bike after a three-hour mountain ride, at halftime during the Super Bowl in which you're *playing,* or whenever you're *being* an athlete.

Tip: To Juice and/or Not to Juice

Many juices offer vital vitamins, minerals, and antioxidants; however, juice can be heavy on calories and simple sugars. Sugars are sugars even when they come from fruit. While I like juices, especially fresh, they should be enjoyed on occasion—not as a several-times-a-day routine.

Check your ingredients to ensure you're getting 100 percent juice and unquestionably without concentrated sugar additives (100 percent natural juice is often sweetened by apple and pear juices, which are still sugars). Also read the serving sizes to see what you're really getting. Amazingly, some juices pack 2.5 servings into a 10- to 12-ounce container. So you look at the label, see the calories and sugars, and forget that it's actually two and a half times that many. Oops!

Minimize your juice intake and try a trick we use around my house: one part juice to about four parts water will make it a reasonable drink. But please don't use juice to replace cool, crisp, clean water.

Tip: "Pop!" Goes the Real Thing

As if you need for me to say this, but here goes: As for the sugar-drenched, preservative-loaded, insulin bottle rockets called soda pop—don't do it. It's little more than a turbocharged "aging potion," nearly perfectly engineered to dehydrate your body. These things are loaded with sugars—and even if it's not the "Prince of Darkness" of sugars, high-fructose corn syrup, it's still pure sugar nonetheless.

As for the "diet" category—I don't mind one now and then myself. If you want a regular soda on occasion, like every leap year or so, fine. Just know that each time you enjoy one it's a little like pounding your head against the wall from the inside—you just don't get any lumps.

Tip: Don't Take No Bull%*$*#

While I'm on the subject, "Don't do it" also covers so-called "energy drinks." Energy? These things are Molotov cocktails loaded with caffeine and sugar. Seriously, it would be difficult for you to drink anything worse! They spike you up and drop you flat, fat, splat! The typical trace elements of nutrients, an amino acid or half a vitamin, are simply window trim.

Tip: Berries are Berry, Berry Good for You

Berries, berries, berries: blueberries, blackberries, raspberries, strawberries, cranberries, and huckleberries are jam-packed with many nutrients and life-enhancing benefits. Berries can protect your brain, your arteries, and other cells in your body from free-radical damage and aging. Not only does sprinkling berries on your salad or cereal make your meal look better, it tastes better too. Fresh organic raspberries, strawberries, or blueberries in a simple vanilla nutrition shake mixed with water can make for an amazing, delicious breakfast treat.

Tip: Set a Tea Time

Tea, especially green tea, is loaded with antioxidants. Green tea has been touted in recent years for its many health benefits in the body and on the brain: reduces cancer rates, enhances mental function, and heightens concentration.

Try enjoying a fine green tea every day—iced in the summer and warm in the winter. Keep an eye out for unnecessary sugars in some bottled versions. All but the finest teas like to dress up the tea with more sugar than you'd want in a drink. I have at least one of my favorites, Tea's Tea, each day. They are free from sugar—just pure, and delicious premium teas.

Tip: Eat Your Omega-3s

The VIP of essential fatty acids is omega-3 (found in certain fish). These fats decrease inflammation, protect against heart disease, blood clots, and strokes. They reduce the risk of Alzheimer's disease, memory loss, and depression. They're found in salmon, herring, mackerel, lake trout, sardines, and some types of white fish. Make it a weekly practice to ensure you're getting an abundance of omega-3s, in addition to other essential fats found in flaxseed, walnuts, and almonds, to name a few.

Tip: Be Happy—Get More Vitamin D

Do you ever wonder why you feel happier on sunny days? It's not just because you're not dealing with rain and cold. When your body absorbs ultraviolet energy from the sun, it converts it into vitamin D. Boost your vitamin D intake with fish such as salmon along with milk fortified with this important vitamin.

Tip: Put Down the Fork

The heaviest people tend to eat fast. Given that it takes nearly 20 minutes for your brain to recognize that your stomach is full, the faster you eat, the more you can stuff yourself. You've done it. I've done it too. We're all guilty of this, especially if eating alone or eating while watching TV. Stop and slow down.

Pay attention to what you're eating and train yourself to take your time. Put down your fork or spoon between each bite.

Tip: Go Nuts!

Nuts can be a healthy, convenient snack and a great addition to many main dishes or salads. They tend to have some protein and fiber, and thanks to the usually healthy fats, they tend to stick to your insides longer than many snacks, helping control blood sugar and appetite. The downside is that they are rich in fats—and thus the calories can quickly add up. When going nuts, try the raw, unsalted variety like almonds, cashews, and walnuts.

Tip: Go Organic

While there's no question organic fruits and vegetables are a nice option, I'm most bullish on organic when it comes to meats and milk products. This is where it is wise to be concerned about hormones. That's why I suggest choosing organic dairy products and selecting your meats from a local butcher you trust.

Tip: Travel Strong

Airports, security, long lines, crowded planes, cranky people, and boxed food. There's little about travel these days that feels like freedom. When you travel, don't set yourself up for the stress and fatigue of being without decent food—set yourself up for success. Take something along to fuel your body and mind so you can arrive strong and alert. I suggest packing some almonds for a snack and water for hydration. My top tip is to pack a shaker bottle and a nutrition shake, like Full Strength, in your carry-on. All you do is add cold water to Full Strength and shake. In one minute you're enjoying a fully energizing shake that will fuel you and keep you going for hours.

Tip: Keep It on the Cob

Corn is fine when it's on the cob or still looks like it could be glued back on—but stay away from its modified cousin, high-fructose corn syrup. You don't need it, don't want it, and you can find volumes of reasons why you should care to avoid it. Keep it out of your food and read your labels, for it's everywhere, even in breads, "natural" sodas, and condiments.

Tip: An Apple a Day

You likely know the old saying, "An apple a day keeps the doctor away." Well, given the state of things in our current medical system and the high emphasis on pharmaceutical solutions, I'm not so sure an apple is going to do it. But an apple is a nearly ideal fruit—it's very low in the glycemic index and has a load of fiber and plenty of vitamins. It's wonderful nutrition, and there is such a delicious variety of apples there's always something new on the next tree. Learn to enjoy an apple nearly every day.

CHAPTER 11

Transformation Training from the Inside Out

Now we've reached the point where it's essential to discuss the specific training strategy you will apply for the next 12 weeks to develop your muscles, shed unwanted body fat, and forge a lean and strong body. In this chapter you will discover that the key to becoming a leaner, stronger *you* is not so much *what* exercises you do—it's not the sets and reps—it's *how* you do them that matters. It's about *form*. It's about *focus*. It's about *intensity.*

When it comes to strength training, I find most people tend to think about the sets, reps, weights, and exercises—the *what,* or *1st Dimension* of strength training. The same applies to cardio conditioning, although here the focal point is typically duration. They give little thought to *how* these sets, reps, and exercises are to be performed—to the *depth* and *quality* of their training.

Believe it or not, a bench press is not just a bench press. A biceps curl is not just a biceps curl. Twenty-five minutes "on the bike" does not necessarily deliver you a stronger, leaner, more vibrant body. Engaging your training with proper form, focus, and intensity can deliver results fast, while simply going through the motions, as most do, will produce only frustration and fatigue.

If two people complete identical exercises, sets and reps, the one who engages the body and mind more fully will produce dramatically greater results. This dimension of quality, the *how,* is what I refer to as the *3rd Dimension of Training.*

How you perform the exercise has more impact than any specific exercise, machine, or even the number of reps. In sports the *how,* often referred to as "intangibles," is the difference between a good athlete and a superstar. Superstars have the physical ability and talent, but more important, they apply their focus and intensity to succeed.

The same is true when it comes to building lean muscle and strength—intensity is key. You must train hard enough to set the growth machinery in motion. Intense effort literally breaks down the muscle on the cellular level, triggering an adaptive response: growth. The greater the intensity generated, the greater the rate of improvement.

Achieving high intensity requires sustained concentration. Staying focused is easier during the first rep, but only those with the most steadfast concentration will reach the highest levels of intensity in their final rep and enjoy the results that follow.

Training at low-intensity levels with a high number of reps simply fatigues the muscles and does little to promote muscle development. Yet this is precisely what so many people who come to strength training with an aerobic conditioning mentality mistakenly do. Believing quantity is king, and unaware of the all important quality of intensity, they go about attempting to squeeze a runner's high out of a dumbbell.

Unfortunately, panting and sweating profusely is not the universal indicator of an "effective" workout. Intensity is a requirement, not an option, for building lean muscle. No amount of low-intensity exercise will effectively promote a lean, shapely, and strong body. On the other hand, if the intensity is high, then a very small amount of training can quickly produce significant results in your muscle tone and strength.

INTENSITY:
THE OTHER HALF OF THE STORY

Typically, intensity is associated with the amount of weight lifted. The heavier the weight, the greater the intensity—the greater the intensity, the greater the alterations in muscle tone and body shape. Thus, you can see why lifting heavy weights could seem to be the answer.

Want bigger biceps? Simply set down the 25s and pick up the 30s—instant intensity! Right? For most, increasing the intensity has meant lifting more weight. While convenient for calculations, this conventional view of intensity is incomplete, it looks outside when intensity is largely generated within. The quality of your training arises from your inner strength. It is much more than the result of the weight being lifted. A dumbbell is, after all, inanimate, serving only to provide resistance. It cannot itself be the *source* of intensity in your muscles.

Focused on the right number of sets and reps or the latest fancy machines, most people's training completely ignores the most critical variable in the strength equation: you! The quality of intensity *you* bring to each and every moment—this 3rd Dimension—is the missing link for so many in training.

In a moment we'll cover the X's and O's for your next 12 weeks, the playbook for your Transformation. It includes the sets, reps, exercises, weekly plan, and everything you need to *do* your Transformation. This sound, effective, and intelligently designed tactical plan, the *what* of Transformation, is the 1st Dimension of Training. In any fitness program you find at the center a common element, the "plan." These plans are often elaborate and complex, as if to support a belief that the plan itself—the sets, reps, and exercises—is the breakthrough. And while most certainly important, the *what* of *Strength for Life* is not the secret to your Transformation success.

The *2nd Dimension of Training*, the *why*, the unstoppable desire to succeed, is what you established in Chapters 6 and 7. All achievement, be it sports, business, or anything else in life, is driven by a compelling desire and an inspiring vision. At this point you should have in place a powerful source of energy that will propel you and keep you moving forward through your Transformation and beyond.

And this brings us to the rarefied air of the 3rd Dimension. You now stand on the threshold of *the secret*—a quantum leap in Transformation—the *how*.

But first the *what*.

For Women Only

The process responsible for muscle growth in women is exactly the same as it is in men. Women can and should train equally as hard as men to reshape their bodies. This includes seeking real strength—not simply trying to make strength training more like cardio exercise.

Without strength training, muscles atrophy. The more muscle you lose, the slower your metabolism works, and that equates to fat storage and weight gain. I cannot stress enough the importance of strength training with intensity. Reflect on Chapter 4 and recall the 7 Wonders of Strength. While all 7 are applicable to women, none may be as relieving to read as the fourth: Muscles Shape You Smaller.

I can understand the fears some women have that strength training will develop big, showy muscles. Many people advocate no less than 15 reps with light weight if you don't want to get "big." Well, that's true, you won't get big on 15 reps, but you won't get anything else either. There will be minimal, if any, improvement in shape. I'm asking you to put any fears aside for the next 12 weeks. Allow the period of Transformation to reshape and energize you as you lose inches where you don't want them and tone your body—the lean muscle you build will translate to the tone and shape you desire.

TRANSFORMATION TRAINING CAMP: SIMPLE, NOT SIMPLISTIC

The *Transformation Training Camp* (TTC) that follows is developed from my more than 20 years of training wisdom—it embodies the integration of simplicity and clarity with the intent of Transformation *and* enjoyment. The TTC focuses on what truly matters most.

The training is neither time-consuming nor complex. It is both maximally effective and efficient for the best results in the least amount of time. A next-level approach to training—accomplished not through intricate, acrobatic maneuvers nor expectations that you give the rest of your life away to train for these next 12 weeks.

Dumbbells are Smart

I designed the *Strength for Life* Transformation program around the use of dumbbells. You can use dumbbells to train all your muscle groups. They offer increased range of motion, require more body-mind synchronization, and keep you naturally focused.

Dumbbells are also safer in many ways than barbells. With dumbbells, you're free to take greater risk, pushing the boundaries of failure sets, without compromising your safety. This a real benefit if you're training without a spotter.

I suggest you use dumbbells for the duration of your Transformation. They are uniquely suited for enhancing focus and training with the FIT practice. You can always choose to swap the dumbbell movements for machines or barbells later. I have included alternative exercises in the back of the book should you elect to do this.

The Weekly Schedule

For the next 12 weeks of the Transformation Training Camp, you follow the same weekly rhythm. Every Monday is a repeat performance of the previous Monday, albeit at an ever-increasing level of strength and stamina. And every Tuesday is the same as the previous, and so forth.

For the TTC you perform three strength training sessions each week—on Mondays, Wednesdays, and Thursdays. The emphasis of training is on *quality* over *quantity*. By applying the Focus Intensity Training system, the *how* (which you will learn about in a moment), your strength training is brief, intense, and challenging.

On Tuesdays and Fridays you experience the classic, proven-effective High-Intensity Interval Training (HIIT) cardio sessions, arguably the most efficient cardio training you can do. A short, invigorating session, HIIT will kick you into another gear in less time than it takes most people to break a sweat during their slow, plodding cardio routines. You also train your abs on these two days, a perfect complement to HIIT.

On Saturdays you enjoy a day of training unlike any other—the Full-Body FIT workout. This is the crescent wrench of training, it's good for just about everything. In this full-body session you strengthen your muscles, improve your stamina, and increase your flexibility while enhancing recovery. The Full-Body FIT engages your muscles, heart, lungs, and mind.

It's the perfect way to end your Transformation week. Here's a look at your *Strength for Life* weekly plan:

7 DAY OVERVIEW

MON	TUES	WED	THURS	FRI	SAT	SUN
STRENGTH	STAMINA	STRENGTH	STRENGTH	STAMINA	FULL BODY	
UPPER-BODY PUSH	HIIT	LOWER-BODY LEGS	UPPER-BODY PULL	HIIT	FIT CIRCUIT	THE 7TH DAY AWAY
Chest Shoulders Triceps Biceps	ABS	Quads Hamstrings Calves	Back Rear-Delts Triceps Biceps	ABS	Strength Stamina Stretch	

Why This Schedule Works

This weekly training schedule is designed to optimize muscle development for your entire body. The three main strength training days are *Push, Legs,* and *Pull.* The names come from the fact that your upper body training is organized around pushing and pulling muscles. The legs day is self-explanatory. The push muscles are your chest, shoulders, and triceps. The pull muscles are your back and biceps. By training these muscle groups in concert, you're maximizing the combined training effect *and* recovery. This way the push and the pull muscles receive ample rest before being trained again.

This routine is also highly advantageous for your legs, providing absolute focus on what is invariably the most challenging of muscle groups to train. Let's face it, most of us would rather clean out the storage space than train legs.

Legs are the most avoided and yet the most important muscle group because of their impact on your body's fat-burning engine and ability to stimulate a positive hormonal environment. When it comes to Transformation, training legs is the Elvis of training—it's the essential foundation.

This schedule is based on science showing that your muscles recover at varying rates—larger muscles take longer to recover from an intense workout than smaller muscles. Regardless of how strong your arms are, arm muscles are smaller than leg muscles. Thus, if you simply trained them both at the same frequency, you would either undertrain your arms or overtrain your legs. That's why on Mondays and Thursdays you're working both your triceps and biceps, because these muscle groups need to be trained more often.

Over the years, I've found this to be a nearly ideal way to balance your total body and optimize your training effectiveness. Plus, while I do enjoy training legs, I also know I am much more inclined to give legs 100 percent when I work them only once per week.

So that's *what* you'll be doing over the course of the next 12 weeks. Now let's turn our attention to the all-important *how.*

Beyond Sets and Reps: The 3rd Dimension of Strength

Multitasking has become so pervasive in our culture that even when people show up at the gym, they bring their mental static with them—their minds are all over the place. Instead of focusing on training, they're thinking about what happened yesterday, planning for the evening ahead, or falling prey to any number of unintended distractions.

This state of commotion undermines the benefits you can derive from training. It's my experience that when people encounter boredom, struggle with motivation, or experience a drop in their progress, they tend to blame the gym, their trainer, or their training program as they absolve themselves from responsibility.

What they're missing out on is an inspiring way to get the most from their precious time training. Focused Intensity Training exchanges these diversions for a deeply enjoyable, highly effective, and optimally efficient way of training.

Focus is the concentration of your attention. It's not necessarily what's on your mind, but *how* you hold your attention without distraction. Focus is not only necessary for effective training, but for performance in all areas of life.

Intensity is the concentration of physical energy—the effort put forth in any moment. It starts with undivided attention; the stronger your focus, the stronger your ability to concentrate energy. Intensity is further amplified by desire, drive, motivation, and will.

To understand how focus and intensity can magnify results, think of a magnifying glass's impact on sunlight. The glass focuses the energy of the sun, creating a beam of intensity (energy) hot enough to ignite a fire. Similarly, focus (your undivided attention) harnesses the intensity (energy in your body) to produce extraordinary results.

The FIT Cycle in Motion

Focus Intensity Training is about creating a rhythm of peak moments of intensity alternating with periods of full recovery in each set. These periods of deep recovery allow you to create higher peaks of focus and intensity. Similarly, the peaks fuel and support a more complete recovery in between each set. This rhythm continues throughout the entire workout.

This *next level* approach to strength training synchronizes your mind and body into a harmonious *flow* state, delivering on its promise of a more enjoyable training experience that's more efficient and effective.

Now we're ready to get into the heart of the FIT cycle, consisting of four techniques used in every set during your training: Ground, Elevate, Focus, and Recover.

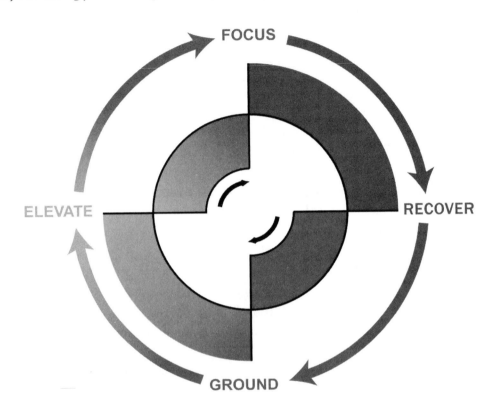

Ground

The FIT cycle begins with the Ground technique. This is the preparation stage for each set. Think of this as home plate, and you're up at bat.

In this stage, which lasts about 15 seconds, breathe normally and connect with your body in a relaxed yet alert posture. Here's where I'd like you to feel gravity's natural pull on your body. Take a moment to notice the ground solidly beneath your feet or the bench beneath you.

Grounding is an effective way to rein in your focus, stop your mind's inner chatter, and set the stage for your set:

I begin by placing my full attention on my breath, making note of the air flowing in and out. I'm enjoying full, even breaths. I pull my awareness into my core, resting my hand on my stomach. Finally, I send my attention down to my feet, feeling the force of gravity and the earth's pull on my body into the bottom of my shoes. This reins in my focus, readying me.

Elevate

Next is the Elevate technique, a series of charging breaths to energize your mind and body just before you begin lifting. Pick up your dumbbells and ready your lifting position. Now breathe into your chest and forcefully expel the air out of your mouth, naturally creating an audible sound. Your inhale should be smooth, controlled, and quick, followed by a fast, powerful exhale. Do this three times in succession. This is your transition from being at rest to catapulting your body into motion.

This breathing technique activates your nervous system and increases the amount of oxygen available to your muscles, creating more energy. *Elevate* is the bridge that takes you from the peace and solidness of *Grounding* to the pinnacle of intensity coming up in *Focus*.

As soon as you've exhaled the third breath, immediately begin the exercise. This is the moment of execution, the act of releasing your strength.

Elevate is a brief but intense, few seconds:

> I pick up my dumbbells and ready myself for my set. I fully inhale through my nose into my chest, then forcefully release the air, blowing out through my mouth, one, two, three . . . a little faster and stronger each time. I'm feeling my energy elevate and start my set immediately upon the third exhale.

Focus

The Focus technique consists of concentrating your attention for high degrees of intensity. Center your attention on the muscles that you're training, both when lifting and lowering the weight. With each rep, draw your attention further into the sensations of the muscles.

As you master this process, your focus will strengthen to a point where all that exists is the immediate sensations within your muscles being trained. It takes practice to develop this type of mental strength; however, every time you engage in a set you're strengthening not only your muscles but your "mental muscle."

With each rep, reach deeper into a state of flow. Generate more focus and intensity, controlling the lifting and lowering of the weight rather than reacting to it. Focus only on the rep at hand, not in pursuit of the final rep of this set. This is a powerful difference even for veterans of strength training.

It's far more effective to contract the muscle and then move the weight, taking the dumbbell along for the ride. Your muscle contracts longer, the intensity is greater, and your results stronger.

The pinnacle of Focus described here may not happen the first time you perform this technique. It starts with the very first rep and lasts throughout the entire set, until the very last moment of your final rep—until you put the weights down:

> I focus my attention on a strong, consistent exhale as I move the weights up for my first repetition, then follow my breath as I steadily inhale and move the weights down. On my next rep, I focus on my form, making sure I execute each movement with extreme precision, maintaining complete control over the dumbbells in my hands.
>
> After a few reps focusing on form, my attention shifts solely to the contractions of the muscles I'm training. With each successive rep, I pull my attention further into the sensations—feeling the heat, intensity, and strength.
>
> I keep channeling my mind into this single-pointed focus, going into the sensations. I'm not thinking about the workout, not even the set I'm doing, my focus is only on the single rep I'm doing right now. If my mind wanders to any other thought, I quickly draw it back to the point of attention.

Recover

Recover is the fourth technique of the FIT cycle. This is where you release the focus and intensity and recover for the next set. *Recovery* is perhaps the most difficult of all the FIT techniques, for it is not something you can *do,* but is something you must allow to happen.

The moment you release the dumbbells you will feel the beginning of this recovery. As your muscles relax, this technique requires you to surrender to this natural movement.

To help deepen this process, find a relaxed, yet alert posture that allows the muscles you've just trained to release additional tension. Then allow your focus to disperse and release so your mind is spacious and relaxed. Finally, allow your breath to drop down into your belly, instead of your chest.

The idea is to actively let go and ride into a deep, quiet, inner rest. Feeling the release of tension, you might experience a descent, as if you're plunging into a pool.

Recovery should last the longest of each of the techniques, about 30 seconds prior to starting your next set with the Ground technique:

> Down go the dumbbells. I've taken my focus into a very tight single point. Now I'm going to let my mind expand, relax, and open before my next set. I drop my breath down into my belly (instead of my chest). I sit down on the edge of the bench, relaxing my body, particularly the muscles I just trained.
>
> This breathing mimics how I naturally breathe when I'm relaxed.
>
> I allow my mind to shift into a broad, open, panoramic stance. My eyes softly gaze, taking in my entire field of vision, no one object comes into sharp focus. If I start to focus on any one object, I take a deep breath and briefly close my eyes. This broad, nonfocal attention allows my focus to take a much needed break.
>
> As my recovery deepens, I stop doing and simply allow myself to be silent, still, at peace.
>
> I don't get caught up in thinking about any one thing. No time for idle chitchat, I'm still engaged in my training. This stage is critical to ready me for my next set. I become the space that allows my thoughts to come and go. After about 30 seconds I'm ready for my next set, slowly transitioning into the Ground stage.

The Space between the Notes

We've talked a lot about the importance of peak focus and intensity in your training; after all, this is where the action is. But there's another side to that coin. It's of equal importance, too often ignored, and hinders people's progress: relaxation and recovery, what I refer to as the "space between the notes."

One of the fundamental laws of physics states, "To every action there is an equal and opposite reaction." This holds true in your training; for every peak in focus and intensity, there must be an equal and opposite recovery. Think of the two points as opposite limits of a child's playground swing. You go forward higher and higher by going farther and farther back. One end activates and amplifies the other. Makes sense, right?

As an example, place this book down and jump. Jump as high as you can and try to touch the ceiling. What steps did you follow?

The first thing you did was recoil, right? Think about it. You actually moved *away* from your goal. You initially brought yourself down toward the ground before you started your ascent. You actually must go down (recover) to go up.

How high would you have jumped if you didn't do this? Try jumping again without recoiling. Your vertical leap (peak) was not as high, was it?

Failing to recognize the equally important dimension of full, spacious recovery limits your peak performance. Your body and mind require this depth of recovery, just as you need sleep each night. Your ability to fully relax and regenerate yourself mentally and physically has a direct impact on your capacity for peak intensity. One does not happen in the absence of the other.

To have the strength for a quality set, you must allow your body to get itself back into a positive energy state—your recovery is as much of the engaged workout as the workout itself. Like the old saying, "the space between the notes creates the music," it's not just the high points, but the moments of recovery that create the harmonious, joyful, flow state of training. Otherwise it would just be noise and not music, or, in our example, just another workout full of drudgery.

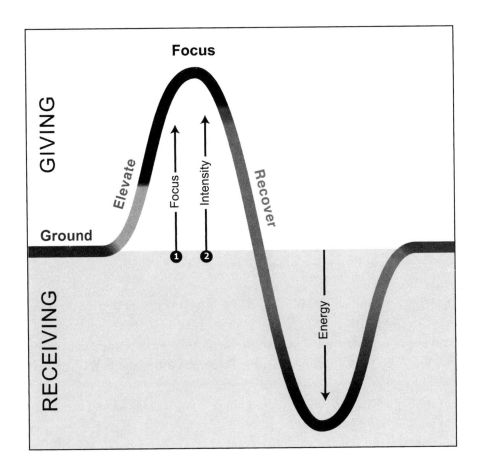

The following image demonstrates a sample FIT sequence with the flow of multiple sets:

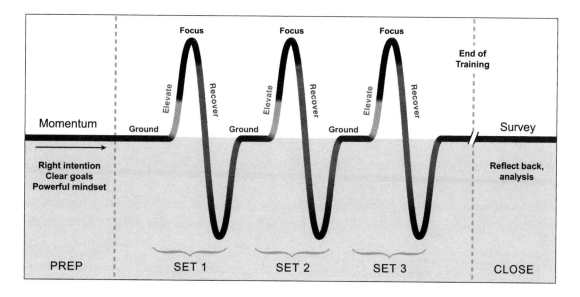

A FIT Discovery

I had been strength training with focus, intensity, and intention for decades, but it wasn't until a few years ago that I recognized its true significance.

In the process of writing *ABSolution: The Practical Solution for Building Your Best Abs,* I hit a block. Frustrated, one afternoon I sat down to talk with my brother Bill about it. I shared all the exercises, sets, and reps. But there was one problem: They were simple workouts—totally, completely, and in every way ordinary. It was baffling. How did I manage to sculpt a world-class set of abs doing the exact same basic exercises that others performed without similar results?

Bill pondered the question and said, "Okay, so what's the secret? What is *the* thing that sets you apart from others?"

After a moment of hesitation, he continued, "It's got to have something to do with that extraordinary degree of focus and intensity you get into in your training."

Something clicked. I could see with great clarity what I had been doing. This was the discovery that strength training is less about the "what"—the sets, the reps, even the exercises—and more about the "how." The *how* produces not only the phenomenal results, but also what makes training an enjoyable practice, with depth, meaning, and impact.

This was, in a moment, the birth of Focus Intensity Training.

This process might sound easy on paper, but don't be discouraged if it's tough at first. It takes practice to master. Once you do, not only will you have a body and strength that reflects your inner mastery, but also the mastery of your mind and focus will be visible in all aspects of your life.

YOUR TRANSFORMATION TRAINING

The Structure of a Set

The first exercise consists of four sets. For the purpose of clarity, a "set" is a series of reps done in succession without rest or setting the weights down.

The first set is 12 reps to get the blood flowing, joints limber, and body and mind alerted to the fact that there's more to follow. That's why I call this the *Salutation* set—it does just that; it's gently calling to your body *and* mind. A sort of ringing of the energetic doorbell, if you will. This should be done with weight you could lift 20 to 25 times.

SET	SET NAME	REP
1	Salutation	12
2	Engagement	10
3	Activation	8
4	Challenge	8+

Next comes a set of 10 reps—the *Engagement* set. This set is the bridge between your warm-up and the intensity to follow. Where the Salutation set is a friendly knock at the door, the Engagement set is more of a fire alarm meant to alert. For these 10 reps, use a weight you could do about 15 times.

The third set is game on—as your muscles are called into full activation with a set of 8 reps. Called the *Activation* set, this is your strength in action. You should use your current best 8-rep max weight, meaning you cannot do one more rep in this set with the weight used.

Your fourth and final set of this exercise is the most intense and demanding so far—hence the reason it's called the *Challenge* set. This set also targets 8 reps with the same weight as the last set; however, now you train to Momentary Muscular Fatigue.

TRAIN TO MOMENTARY MUSCULAR FATIGUE

Training to Momentary Muscular Fatigue provides the single most effective way to produce gains in muscular strength and reshape your body. This holds true for both men and women.

This type of fatigue occurs when you can no longer move the weight up. This does not mean you can use sloppy form as your muscles begin to tire. Rather, it means that you lift a weight as many times with proper form. You test this during your Challenge sets.

Training to the point of Momentary Muscular Fatigue is not easy. While it can provide optimal benefits in minimal time, it requires considerable mental and physical effort—at times exceeding a person's ability. Consequently, there may be instances where it is not warranted (yet). These include:

- Beginners. If you're a beginner, I encourage you to learn the proper mechanics, breathing, and mental focus prior to training to *fatigue*. And use a spotter for safety.
- Non-Transformation Training. During times of down-training, recovery, or preparation, such as the Base Camp phase—or any times where a reduction in training demands is needed to promote recovery.
- Athletes. If you're an athlete who trains intensely outside the gym, it may be best to avoid training to *fatigue*, or include it in the appropriate phase of your off-season training.

FOCUS INTENSITY INDEX

Success in strength training is often mistakenly measured strictly by the amount of weight lifted. By this point you know it takes more than a dumbbell. While the weight is a factor, focus and intensity—the sum total of the *mental* and *physical* effort put forth in any moment—are the primary ingredients for generating change in your body. And as your muscles move only when your mind commands them, strength begins on the inside—and is the product of willful, concentrated effort.

I'm a firm believer that what gets measured gets done. In the absence of a measure of performance—a gauge for intensity—there is no feedback and thus no improvement. This wisdom applies to your training as much as it does in business and in life. For you to consistently

The Baseball Toss

If you throw a baseball as hard as you can, how fast would it go? No idea? Me either, but I can assure you of one thing: If a speed gun measures your throw, your second throw would be faster, and your third faster still. This is the nature of feedback—the instant we measure ourselves, we seek to improve. This underscores the strength of the connection between your body and mind.

> ## Cut a Deeper Groove
>
> A commonly used practice is a "pyramid" style set structure—where the number of reps decrease with each set, like 12-10-8-6, and then increase again with sets of 8, 10, or 12. This can be a very effective way to train, but the advantage of doing two consecutive sets with the same weight and number of reps, as you do in the TTC, allows you to gauge your strength on the first set and then cut a deeper groove with more focus and intensity on your second.
>
> The 12-10-8-8 pattern is like getting a second tee shot, a do-over. The second "8" is almost always a truer, deeper reflection of your capacity.

achieve peak levels of intensity—the effort necessary to produce and improve over time—you must both define and measure it.

This desire is the inspiration for the *Focus Intensity Index*. It's a way to place a relative measure on your intensity levels that allows you to consistently achieve and improve upon them.

The Focus Intensity Index is a simple tool that has worked well for my clients and myself over the decades—a clarifying 1 to 5 rating scale. Each set in the TTC program prescribes a corresponding target level of intensity. The more challenging the set, the higher the level of intensity required. Here's a look at the Focus Intensity Index levels:

Level 1: Pre-Workout Warm-up

This is the lowest perceptible level of intensity. It's any willful movement of your body that you can actually feel. Your five-minute, low-intensity, pre-workout warm-up is a Level 1.

Level 2: Salutation Sets

Level 2 is the entry point for weight lifting of any sort. There's resistance but it's not challenging and does not require much effort. Your Salutation sets are targeted for Level 2.

Level 3: Engagement Sets

Now you're entering into the realm of exertion—you can feel the weight. Here your mental state and focus are engaged. You are activating the muscle without running out of steam and power. Your Engagement sets are targeted for Level 3.

Level 4: Activation Sets

This is where the going gets tough. At this level your mental focus is every bit as important as your physical potential—and for many *the* limiting factor. If you're able to reach and sustain this level, it will feel as if you completed the necessary reps but with little room to spare. You might have been able to do one or two more reps, but it requires significant levels of focus and intensity to complete a Level 4 set. Your Activation sets are targeted for Level 4.

Level 5: Challenge and Drop Sets

The magical moment when a muscle is producing as much force as it is capable of is your *Peak Intensity*. It requires absolute focus and total effort. To reach this esteemed level of intensity often requires reaching total muscle fatigue, or pushing beyond previous limits where part of you may have wanted to back out. You may have started out to complete 8 reps and failed at 6 or reached 9, but either way, you reached your absolute Peak Intensity. Your Challenge sets and Drop sets are targeted for Level 5.

In your Tracking Forms for each workout you will see a + next to your target number of reps, indicating you will take the set to Momentary Muscular Fatigue.

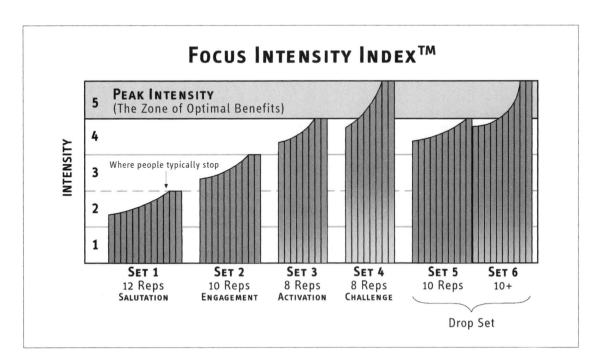

Intensity Always Rises

Let me illustrate an all-out Level 5 set of the dumbbell bench press, the first set calling forth the Peak Intensity on your Monday workout. My target is eight reps with 80-pound dumbbells.

On the first rep I feel strong. I press it up smooth and solid, with ease. The question, "Should I have gone heavier?" flashes through my mind. Before this first rep I held a full reserve of strength. After completing it, there's a certain loss of strength.

My strength is still high, keeping the intensity moderate. With each successful rep, the intensity of effort and concentration of energy in my chest muscles elevate quickly. By the seventh rep the tension has gone from burning to scorching hot; this is where a novice lifter might call it off. But I'm accustomed to this intensity, and it's actually enhancing my focus. The weight is no longer moving quickly, but it is moving smoothly. My confidence is bolstered as I reach the uppermost point of the eighth rep—where I take an extended pause to regroup and summon my inner strength.

Though the last rep was a challenge, I'm not done yet. I think only, "One more," nothing else enters my mind. Lowering the weight for the ninth rep, one above my target, I'm focused. It's the strictest, most controlled descent yet. My chest is charging with energy on the way down. Reaching the low point, I pause the dumbbells for a fraction of a second before I release my full force. Driving the dumbbells up takes everything I've got. It's not an explosive force, but the weight is moving steady and strong, one inch at a time. There's no assurance I'm getting this one up, but when it begins to move a little stronger, faster, I know I've got it; although to see my body quake you'd not be too sure. I complete the ninth rep and put down the dumbbells, knowing this is the Peak Intensity—a Level 5.

Had I been capable of doing one or two more reps and quit, I'd have fallen short of Peak Intensity. Had I chosen a weight I could have done for only six reps but stopped at three, I'd have come up short of Peak Intensity too.

Intensity increases in this fashion across a set from the first repetition to the last. At the beginning there exists 100 percent strength in reserve of what is possible. For example, after completing the first of my targeted eight repetitions, there was a loss of a certain measure of strength. The demands increased from repetition to repetition as my set progressed. Thus, it required greater effort to complete each repetition as my capacity to generate muscular strength decreased. The ninth rep was my most difficult, requiring higher levels of intensity than all previous reps. My Peak Intensity was achieved during the final repetition, when Momentary Muscular Fatigue occurred, in this example, my ninth rep.

Tracking Your Progress

To produce your most significant results, to stimulate the most change, you must both gauge and track your focus and intensity. In your Workout Tracking Form there's a column with your Target Intensity Level (TIL) for each set. Intensity, as the measure of *effort* for any rep or over the course of a set, is subjective. Record your *Actual* Intensity Level following each set in the space provided.

As you press into your potential over the course of your Transformation, you will continually discover a greater capacity to exhibit strength and harness focus—thus raising your relative levels of intensity. For example, those new to the sensations of muscle fatigue may reach their *perceived* Peak Intensity well before Momentary Muscular Fatigue—and stop. Beginners tend to have a lower tolerance because they are not used to intense training and may not have the adaptive skills to exert high levels of effort. This is okay and can be expected as part of the process. Intermediate and advanced trainers tend to have greater ability to activate their muscles, and as a result will experience their Level 5 differently than a beginner.

Throughout this training I refer to the Focus Intensity Index as common language you and I now share—so when I say, "This set is to be performed at intensity Level 5," you know what that means—*for you*.

DAILY GUIDE TO FULL STRENGTH

Following is a day-by-day overview for your training. Be sure to maintain proper form. In Appendix D, I've included detailed instructions, along with photos of every exercise you perform in the TTC. Please take the time to review these, even if you're already familiar with them. Bring some new precision to your training—and if you're new to any or all of them, use this guide over and over to elevate your technique and improve your form. Also, you may consider enlisting a qualified professional trainer to help you develop and refine your training.

A Tracking Form is provided for each workout.

First, Warm-up

Before you jump into your strength training sessions, invest five minutes warming up your body with some form of low-intensity cardio. Cold muscles are fragile. As you pump blood into your muscles, warming them, they become much more elastic. Do just enough work to begin to perspire.

Monday: Upper-Body Strength Push

Ah, Monday, the start of a new week. Hopefully renewed and refreshed from the weekend, you'll hit the ground running. And in my view, there's no better way than starting your Transformation week with the Push day, feeling your own power of pushing into the world and moving forward with strength. The emphasis of your training is on the chest, shoulders, and triceps. These are your muscles that push up, off, and out.

After a warm-up, you begin by training your largest, strongest push muscles: the chest. The selected exercises are the dumbbell bench press, four sets, followed by two sets of dumbbell flyes, one of which is a drop set (see below).

You start with the Salutation set, a 12-rep strength warm-up, a greeting to your muscles. The next set is the Engagement set of 10 reps. This set, a little more demanding, engages your muscles and mind—preparing for the intensity of the next few sets. The third set, Activation, is your first 8-rep set, leading you to the crème de la crème, the pinnacle of the dumbbell bench press, the Challenge set, your final 8 reps, which you take to total Momentary Muscular Fatigue.

The Magic of the Drop Set

A drop set is the second of two sets of the same exercise, done in rapid succession, with no rest in between. It's one set done to the point when you can no longer complete a quality rep without cheating in some fashion. Then you set the dumbbells down, pick up lighter weights, and repeat. The time between sets is only what's necessary to change the weights. The second set is performed with about 50 to 70 percent of the previous weight, hence the term "drop," which refers to a drop in the weight.

By not allowing your muscles to recuperate between sets of the same exercise, the intensity and demands on the muscle continue to escalate (even though the second set is done with lighter weight). Drop sets take you beyond the normal limits, testing your heart, desire, and will from a place so deep inside that one rarely visits; and it is very effective for building strength.

The next two sets are dumbbell flyes. The first set is 10 reps, followed, without rest, by a second set of 10 reps. This is called a drop set.

After the chest, you train your shoulders, focusing on the front and side of your deltoid muscles with four sets of dumbbell side lateral raises. You follow the same progression of intensity as previous; however, you perform 12-10-10-8 as your shoulders respond better to these rep ranges. The last set is a drop set. Side lateral raises are an excellent lift for giving the shoulders shape while safely increasing strength.

Next you train your triceps and biceps (the only nonpush muscles you work today). Each exercise—triceps kickbacks and biceps curls—follows a 12-10-8-8 rhythm; the last set in each is a drop set.

Following your day's training, take a few minutes to do the Post-Workout 1-2-3 (see following). And then it's time for some much-needed nourishment to jump-start your recovery—and lock in the gains.

Don't Shoulder This Burden

Your foot has 26 bones, your hand has a crazy opposable thumb that enables you to do all sorts of things. Yet my vote for the most extraordinary construct of our bodies is the shoulder. It's the most flexible, versatile, and oft-used joint in our bodies. And, if you're not impressed, one look at the inner workings will change all that: a free-floating ball pressed against a custom-fit landing pad held in place by 17 muscles.

While the shoulder's architecture is amazing, its foundation is not the most sound. It's not all that difficult to knock out, break down, or injure. And even if you have no appreciation for the king of all joints, injure your shoulder just one time, as I have, and you'll spend a lifetime guarding it.

You may have noticed that the TTC workout does not include any of the classic, often standard overhead presses. This is not by accident. I find that the risk-to-benefit ratio does not justify them. Now, I'm not suggesting that if you press a weight over your head you're bound to end up injured. The risk, however, is ever present, the price of injury high, and the upside to doing these lifts small.

Worry not about undertraining your shoulders. They receive ample work in the TTC, indirectly during chest training, which highly recruits from shoulder muscles/front deltoids, and directly via side lateral raises (side deltoids) and reverse flyes (rear deltoids).

In my view, the primary reason overhead presses remain such a staple lift is because they are part of the lifting archetype that has been passed down for generations like an old wives' tale. It's what seems logical—it looks like what the shoulder is supposed to do. Press things up.

Unless you're a pro athlete trying to make the team, there are many other ways to shape and strengthen your shoulders without the increased risk inherent in performing the shoulder press. My advice is simple: Just don't do them.

Monday *Shawn* **PUSH** Chest | Shoulders | Triceps + Biceps

DATE _June 23_ WK# _____7_____ START TIME _6:30_ FINISH TIME _7:07 AM_

	SET	EXERCISE	TBS	PLANNED WEIGHT/REPS	TiL	ACTUAL WEIGHT/REPS	AiL
CHEST	1	Dumbbell Bench Press		50 /12	2	50 / 12	2
	2		60	60 /10	3	60 / 10	3
	3		60	70 /8	4	70 / 8	4
	4		60	80 /8+	(5)	80 / 7	(5)
	5	Dumbbell Flyes	60	55 /10	4	55 / 10	4
	6		0	40 /10+	(5)	40 / 11	(5)
SHOULDERS	7	Dumbbell Side Raises	60	15 /12	2	15 / 12	2
	8		60	20 /10	3	20 / 10	3
	9		60	30 /10	4	30 / 10	4
	10		0	20 /8+	(5)	20 / 9	(5)
ARMS	11	Dumbbell Triceps Kickbacks	60	20 /12	2	20 / 12	2
	12		60	30 /10	3	30 / 10	3
	13		60	35 /8	4	35 / 7	(5)
	14		0	20 /8+	(5)	20 / 8	(5)
	15	Dumbbell Biceps Curls	60	30 /12	2	30 / 12	2
	16		60	35 /10	3	35 / 10	3
	17		60	45 /8	4	45 / 9	4
	18		0	30 /8+	(5)	30 / 10	(5)

POST-WORKOUT ❶ RECORD ❷ PROJECT ❸ REFLECT

I increased my strength significantly on my DB side raises!
I could have gotten more on sets 17 & 18, STAY FOCUSED!

★ = DROP-SET   + = TO FAILURE SET |TBS| = TIME *BEFORE* SET (Secs) |TiL| = TARGET INTENSITY LEVEL |AiL| = ACTUAL INTENSITY LEVEL

Wednesday: Lower-Body Strength (Legs)

Wednesday—the center and peak of the week. Get through this and it's downhill to the weekend.

You'll be quick to notice I placed legs, traditionally the most challenging of workout days and also the most rewarding, smack-dab in the middle of the week. Why? For one, it works. It's the perfect way to split your two upper-body training days. And second, beyond all technical reasons, what for many may be the best reason of all—for the weekend warrior. Training legs, your body's largest collection of muscles, can take a lot out of you. By training legs on Wednesday you'll be back at strength and ready to engage in nearly any activity you want to by the weekend.

Leg training is much more about effectiveness and *quality* of movement. By using perfect form and deeply focusing on the muscles, you will get an amazing, effective leg workout without risking your back.

First, you execute two exercises that engage all the major muscles in your legs (glutes, quads, hamstrings, calves): dumbbell lunges and dumbbell squats. Dumbbell lunges open your leg workout with the 12-10-8-8 rhythm introduced on Monday.

The next two sets are dumbbell squats. The first set is 10 reps followed by a drop set of 10.

Next you're going to challenge your hamstrings with dumbbell straight-leg deadlifts. This exercise, if done incorrectly, can strain your back, so please pay attention to proper form. Start with lighter weights and work your way up safely. You follow the 12-10-8-8 pattern, with the last 8 reps performed as a drop set. The next two sets are *sumo squats* performed as a drop set. The first set is 12 reps, followed, without rest, by a second set of 12 reps.

The exercises above all engage your glutes—the much admired muscles of the rear end, so essential for shaping.

You finish up the Wednesday workout with dumbbell single-leg calf raises. Your calves did a significant amount of work already during the lunges, squats, and deadlifts. This exercise is done continuously, with no rest. But because you're alternating legs, one leg is resting while the other one is working. Perform four sets of 12 reps each.

As difficult as this day can be at first, once you develop your FIT practice and fully embrace this workout, my bet is you will find this your favorite. For me, it's the most invigorating for my body. It leaves me with an unparalleled sense of accomplishment each time I train.

Thursday: Upper-Body Strength Pull

This day is very much like your Monday, in that you perform five exercises in a similar pattern of sets and reps—except your training is focused on the muscles responsible for pulling, including your back and biceps.

Why Thursday? You have not trained your upper body since Monday, so it's ready and it doesn't affect your readiness for the Full-Body FIT Saturday training.

Your back is the second largest collection of muscles on your body, second only to your legs. That means there's much to train and much to gain from training it well.

Once again, using dumbbell exercises only, you start with four sets of one-arm dumbbell rows in the familiar 12-10-8-8 pattern. This is followed by two sets of 10 dumbbell pullovers, the second set a drop set.

Next you work rear deltoids (back of your shoulders) with reverse flyes. Because you're working the shoulders, you follow the 12-10-10-8 sequence with lighter weights that allow you to focus on form and fully contract muscles.

And finally, you finish this day much as you did Monday—with arms. First your four sets of seated dumbbell curls, and then closing strong with four sets of dumbbell triceps kickbacks. Both sets follow the 12-10-8-8, with a drop set closing out each exercise.

Tuesday and Friday: High-Intensity Interval Training and Abs (HIIT)

A strong heart and efficient lungs are an important part of what your body needs to function at full strength, and that's what Tuesdays and Fridays are about. You'll also strengthen your core with the Transformation abs routine.

For years I struggled with low-intensity, time-consuming, mind-numbing cardio exercise. As intolerable as it was for me, it was the accepted method for shedding excess fat. This all changed in 1996 when I discovered the science of *High Intensity Interval Training,* or HIIT, a highly effective form of cardio training specifically designed to maximize fat loss and minimize time without cannibalizing lean muscle.

Whether you're a longtime endurance athlete, a cardio fanatic, avoid cardio at all costs, or fall somewhere in between, HIIT is the right cardio training for your best Transformation. It can help you reshape your body and make your strength visible for all to see.

The premise of HIIT is simple: Rather than waste time exercising at a slow pace, hoping fat melts off before you're overcome with boredom, you alternate intervals of moderate-intensity cardio training with short bursts of near maximum effort. These intervals keep you focused and engaged.

Since its discovery, HIIT is *the* cardio-training program I use myself, share with clients, and describe in my writing, seminars, and conversations. HIIT is now the standard cardiovascular training method for Transformation.

In research, HIIT has repeatedly outperformed conventional forms of low-intensity cardio. It expends more calories, not only while you're training, but for hours afterward. That's right, while you're relaxing, eating, working at your desk, and even sleeping, your metabolism races

Wednesday *Shawn*   **LEGS**   Quads | Hamstrings | Calves

DATE *June 25* WK# *7*   START TIME *6:00* FINISH TIME *6:41 AM*

	SET	EXERCISE	TBS	PLANNED WEIGHT/REPS	TiL	ACTUAL WEIGHT/REPS	AiL
LEGS/QUADS	1	Dumbbell Step Lunges		45 /12	2	45 / 12	2
	2		60	55 /10	3	55 / 10	3
	3		60	60 /8	4	60 / 8	4
	4		60	65 /8+	(5)	65 / 7	(5)
	5	Dumbbell Squats	60	75 /10	4	75 / 9	(5)
	6		0	50 /10+	(5)	50 / 11	(5)
HAMSTRINGS	7	Dumbbell Straight-Leg Deadlifts	60	40 /12	2	40 /12	2
	8		60	45 /10	3	45 /10	3
	9		60	50 /8	4	50 /10	4
	10		0	55 /8+	(5)	55 /10	(5)
	11	Dumbbell Sumo Squats	60	100 /12	4	100 /10	4
	12		0	70 /12+	(5)	70 / 9	(5)
CALVES	13	Dumbbell Single-Leg Calf Raises	60	65 /12	2	65 / 12	2
	14		0	70 /12	3	70 / 12	3
	15		0	75 /12	4	75 / 12	4
	16		0	75 /12+	(5)	75 / 14	(5)

POST-WORKOUT ❶ RECORD   ❷ PROJECT   ❸ REFLECT

Increase my weight to 60 lbs on last set of deadlifts.
Lower weight to 65 on set 12/Sumo Squats next week.

★ = DROP-SET   + = TO FAILURE SET |TBS| = TIME *BEFORE* SET (Secs) |TiL| = TARGET INTENSITY LEVEL |AiL| = ACTUAL INTENSITY LEVEL

STRENGTH FOR LIFE WORKOUT TRACKER

Thursday *Shawn* | **PULL** | Back | Rear Delts | Triceps + Biceps

DATE *June 26* WK# *7*   START TIME *6:20* FINISH TIME *6:59 AM*

SET	EXERCISE	TBS	PLANNED WEIGHT/REPS	TiL	ACTUAL WEIGHT/REPS	AiL
BACK 1	One-Arm Dumbbell Rows		50 /12	2	50 / 12	2
2		60	60 /10	3	60 / 10	3
3		60	70 /8	4	70/ 8	4
4		60	80 /8+	(5)	80 / 10	(5)
5	Dumbbell Pullovers	60	65 /10	4	65 / 10	3
6	★	0	40 /10+	(5)	40 / 15	4
SHOULDERS 7	Reverse Dumbbell Flyes	60	15 /12	2	15 / 12	2
8		60	20 /10	3	20/ 10	3
9		60	25 /10	4	25/ 10	4
10	★	0	15 /8+	(5)	15 / 9	(5)
ARMS 11	Lying Dumbbell Triceps Extensions	60	25 /12	2	25 / 12	2
12		60	35 /10	3	35 / 10	3
13		60	40 /8	4	40 / 10	4
14	★	0	25 /8+	(5)	25 / 10	(5)
15	Dumbbell Biceps Curls	60	30 /12	2	30 / 12	2
16		60	40 /10	3	40 / 10	3
17		60	45 /8	4	45 / 8	4
18	★	0	30 /8+	(5)	30 / 9	(5)

POST-WORKOUT   **1** RECORD   **2** PROJECT   **3** REFLECT

Increase the weight on set #4. Try 85's next week.

Not the right weight – Bring more intensity on sets 5&6.

★ = DROP-SET   + = TO FAILURE SET |TBS| = TIME *BEFORE* SET (Secs) |TiL| = TARGET INTENSITY LEVEL |AiL| = ACTUAL INTENSITY LEVEL

The Transformation of Cardio Training

Research in the 1960s brought the positive impact of regular cardiovascular training to our attention. With its capacity for improving the functioning of our heart and lungs, and overall positive impacts on health, cardio quickly became the way to "get in shape."

In the 1970s the jogging boom was in full swing. The 1980s featured leg warmers, spandex, and headbands as aerobics caught fire. And with it, the promise of cardio exercise grew beyond heart and lungs to include everything from a leaner, more toned body to a more vibrant person in every way.

The 1990s delivered cardio kickboxing and spin classes. And in many ways this myth of aerobic exercise as an all-purpose workout persists today. And why not? Whether it's running the road, spinning in a gym, or kicking it up to a rhythmic beat, the arms and legs are in motion and sweat is pouring, which must mean calories are burning, fat is dissolving. Thus we assume, "This must be *the way* to get in shape."

And, indeed, improved cardiovascular functioning *is* an important part of being in shape. Yet, the promise that somehow a heart that pumps stronger and improved lung capacity makes a body stronger or more shapely is erroneous.

Millions of people each year are drawn to low-intensity cardio as an easy, nonthreatening way to shape up. And millions annually fail to realize significant or lasting change. While anything that increases a person's activity is positive, you cannot ignore that for decades low-intensity cardio has been packaged with a suite of promises it simply cannot deliver.

Not only does extended sessions of cardio fail to enhance muscle, tone, or shape—it's a well-established scientific fact that endurance-based cardio is actually in opposition to the vital lean muscle you're so meticulously seeking to sculpt during your Transformation. Thus, should you choose to engage in low-intensity, long-duration cardio during your TTC, you will effectively be taking a giant eraser to your precious gains in lean muscle earned in your strength training sessions.

---

along at an elevated rate long after you've finished. More calories burned equals *more fat lost—up to 50 percent.* When it comes to transforming lives, HIIT is the perfect fit.

A HIIT for Your Transformation

One of the aspects of the *Strength for Life* HIIT Cardio program that people tell me they like most is that it can be applied to all sorts of activities, in or out of the gym. I like to apply HIIT when running stairs or short sprints, but it can be done as effectively on nearly any cardio machine or activity where you can alternate periods of high intensity with periods of low intensity.

Start by engaging in a 3-minute warm-up. Take a gradual stepped approach to ready your body before reaching for your highest levels of intensity. Then begin your first interval with 60 seconds at high intensity before returning to a lower level of intensity for 60 seconds. This allows you to catch your breath and prepare for your next all-out assault. Drop the little red dots on the machine to about 30 to 40 percent of your peak (on a scale of 1 to 10, you're at a 3 or 4). Continue this pattern of alternating high-intensity and low-intensity 60-second intervals for a series of 8 peaks. After your last peak interval, enjoy a 2-minute low-intensity cool-down. This ends your HIIT workout.

Your time limit is 20 minutes. If you give yourself more time, you'll naturally reduce your intensity in order to fill it. So don't do it. Stick with 20 minutes and make every minute count. Stay engaged in your training and don't allow a newspaper, magazine, or TV to distract you.

Depending upon your condition at the outset of your Transformation, you may need to adjust the intensity of your peaks. It's up to you to discover your upper limits. All peaks are not created equal. At your high-intensity levels you should be pushing yourself to make it the full 60 seconds. If during the high-intensity intervals you are not resisting the desire to turn it down during the final 10 to 15 seconds, you're not at your upper limits.

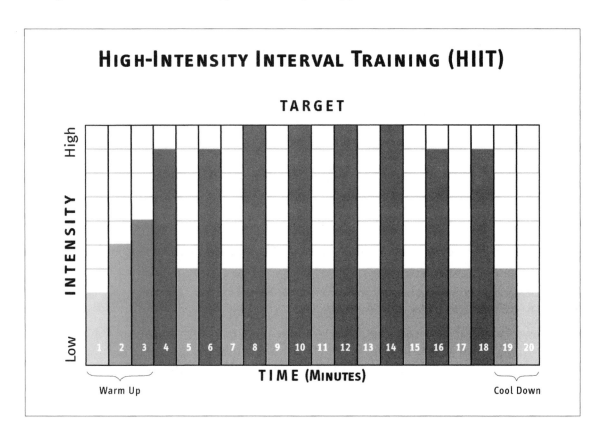

My personal favorite machine in the gym for HIIT is the stair-stepper; however, HIIT can also be readily applied to the stationary bicycle, treadmill, rowing machine, elliptical, or nearly any cardio equipment. Each machine has its own way of stepping up the pace and/or resistance, so take the time to learn how to properly adjust the equipment of your choice. It's important to know that your peak is when you're maxed out, not when the machine is being maxed out.

HIIT'n the Track

When taking HIIT outside—be it to the track, the stairs, the sand, or even a jump rope—it's the same theory, although you can measure your intervals with time, distance, or by count. When sprinting or running stairs, the intensity can get high quickly. If you haven't tried to sprint since you were a kid, you're in for a shock. If you take off like you're being timed for a 40-yard dash, you may find yourself scoring a "9-1-1."

Intervals tend to be more strenuous outside than on the best cardio machines. For this reason, rather than 60-second intervals, I advise starting with 30-second high-intensity intervals when applying HIIT at the track. You may choose a 30-second all-out sprint to get as far around the track as you can before coming to a slow jog or walk. This will get you as far as 30 seconds of sprinting will get you—be that halfway around a quarter-mile track or half that.

You may try sprinting for 20, 40, or even 100 yards. Then follow the sprint by at least an equal distance of walking as you catch your breath. On the stairs or jump rope, I like to set a target for a number of stairs or jumps and count off as I'm going. The shorter intervals allow you to reach higher intensity safely. It's not a contest. It's about you finding and pushing *your* limits.

Let's HIIT It!

High-Intensity Interval Training will test you and you will be stronger for its challenge. Although you should ultimately strive to push yourself to run near your maximum, you will want to adjust and develop at your own pace, according to your level of cardiovascular fitness. Whatever works best for you, find your peaks and keep your cardio training to 20 minutes.

Focus on getting the most out of each high-intensity interval one at a time, expanding your stamina and generating the greatest metabolic boost for your transforming body.

Abs

Following your HIIT cardio, it's time to address your core: abs.

Much like your strength training workouts, your ab training is brief and intense; not the typical rep-athon you may encounter at the gym. These exercises are not speed movements, instead they are slow, intense contractions of your abs that, when done properly, can and should burn.

You perform three ab exercises, beginning with Swiss Ball ab crunches. Next up is reverse crunches. Finally, you finish with ab crunches. Each exercise is performed for three sets of 12–15 repetitions, with about a 30-second rest between each set. A good rule of thumb is if you can perform more than 15 reps in any one set, you're not bringing a sufficient level of intensity to effect change in your physique.

As with all exercises in the *Strength for Life* program, detailed descriptions are provided in Appendix D.

Saturday: Full-Body FIT

Saturdays are your day for a challenging, energizing, and renewing session—something new. A *fully integrated* training experience that will engage your *strength,* enhance your *stamina,* and *stretch* your body.

Your Saturday training is an integrated hybrid of both cardio and strength conditioning bolstered by vital stretch training. It's an enjoyable, quick-paced, challenging, and mindful workout boosting you by activating every major muscle in your body, elevating your metabolism, and flushing out toxins.

This style of training differs from your foundational strength training workouts Monday, Wednesday, and Thursday. Its fresh approach puts a wrap on your week, but please don't make the mistake of thinking it's optional. It's as important to your Transformation as any workout in the schedule.

There are two parts to this workout: first, a circuit-style strength training regimen; and second, a series of stretches designed to increase flexibility. The dumbbells' version of the strength circuit takes 15 to 20 minutes to complete. Stretching is about 12 minutes. Altogether this day comes in at about 35 minutes—a perfect workout to close your Transformation week.

FIT Strength Circuit

Following your standard five-minute warm-up, you start the first of two to three circuits consisting of six different strength exercises. The six exercises in the following chart are performed in succession, with little to no rest in between, for 15 reps each.

Once you complete one circuit (all six exercises), you rest before beginning your second circuit. Rather than completing the FIT cycle with each set, this circuit challenges you to maintain a steady (and even elevated) degree of focus over a longer period. Even though you use much lighter weight than on your Challenge sets during the week, the cumulative effect of 15 reps in consecutive sets builds, resulting in a high degree of intensity by the final rep of each circuit.

It's here, at this high point where the full FIT cycle (and deep recovery) is initiated. The

Tuesday *Shawn*

HIIT/ABS

HIIT | ABS

DATE *June 24* WK# *7* START TIME *6:10* FINISH TIME *6:45 AM*

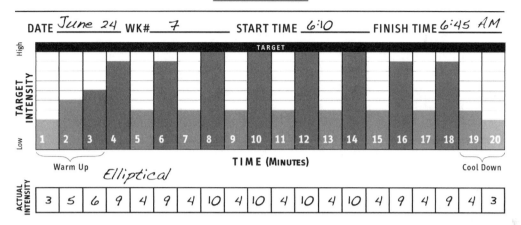

Warm Up — *Elliptical* — TIME (MINUTES) — Cool Down

ACTUAL INTENSITY	3	5	6	9	4	9	4	10	4	10	4	10	4	10	4	9	4	9	4	3

	SET	EXERCISE	PLANNED REPS	ACTUAL REPS
ABS	1	Swiss Ball Ab Crunches (30 Seconds Rest Between Sets)	12–15	15
	2		12–15	15
	3		12–15	14
	4	Reverse Crunches (30 Seconds Rest Between Sets)	12–15	15
	5		12–15	13
	6		12–15	14
	7	Cross Crunches (30 Seconds Rest Between Sets)	12–15	15
	8		12–15	12
	9		12–15	15

POST-WORKOUT   ❶ RECORD   ❷ PROJECT   ❸ REFLECT

HIIT: Reached new peak. On track for personal best.
Core work brings my whole body to life.

HIIT/ABS

Friday *Shawn*   HIIT | ABS

DATE _June 27_ WK# _____7_____ START TIME _6:00_ FINISH TIME _6:35 AM_

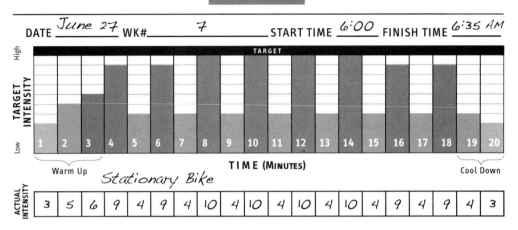

TARGET INTENSITY — High / Low

TIME (Minutes)

Warm Up   *Stationary Bike*   Cool Down

ACTUAL INTENSITY

3	5	6	9	4	9	4	10	4	10	4	10	4	10	4	9	4	9	4	3

SET	EXERCISE	PLANNED REPS	ACTUAL REPS
1	Ab Crunches (30 Seconds Rest Between Sets)	12–15	15
2		12–15	15
3		12–15	13
4	Reverse Crunches (30 Seconds Rest Between Sets)	12–15	15
5		12–15	14
6		12–15	12
7	Cross Crunches (30 Seconds Rest Between Sets)	12–15	15
8		12–15	15
9		12–15	15

ABS

POST-WORKOUT   **1** RECORD   **2** PROJECT   **3** REFLECT

Great way to end the week. Abs feel great.

Saturday *Shawn* **FIT CIRCUIT** Total Body

DATE *June 28* WK# *7* START TIME *7:30* FINISH TIME *8:07 AM*

	EXERCISE	TiL	CIRCUIT 1 WEIGHT/REP	AiL	CIRCUIT 2 WEIGHT/REP	AiL	CIRCUIT 3 WEIGHT/REP	AiL
1	Dumbbell Bench Press	3	50 / 15	3	50 / 15	3	50 / 15	3
2	One-Arm Dumbbell Row	3	50 / 15	3	50 / 15	3	50 / 15	3
3	Dumbbell Side Raises	3	15 / 15	3	15 / 15	3	15 / 15	3
4	Lying Dumbbell Triceps Extensions	4	25 / 15	4	25 / 15	4	25 / 15	4
5	Biceps Curls	4	25 / 15	4	25 / 15	4	25 / 15	4
6	Sidestep Lunges	4	15 / 15	4	15 / 15	4	15 / 15	4

FIT CIRCUIT

No rest between each exercise. 2–3 minute recovery between circuits. 3rd set is optional.

	EXERCISE	TARGET DURATION	ACTUAL DURATION
1	Toe Touches	30–60 Seconds	*60 seconds*
2	Lunge (each side)	30–60 Seconds	*60 seconds/side*
3	Flye Stretch (each side)	30–60 Seconds	*60 seconds/side*
4	Twists (each side)	30–60 Seconds	*60 seconds/side*
5	Seal Stretch	30–60 Seconds	*60 seconds*
6	Cat Stretch	30–60 Seconds	*60 seconds*

FIT STRETCH

POST-WORKOUT ❶ RECORD ❷ PROJECT ❸ REFLECT

26 Minutes in Circuits, 11 min. stretches.
Feels Great! Body open and flexible.

|TiL| = TARGET INTENSITY LEVEL |AiL| = ACTUAL INTENSITY LEVEL

Peak Intensity reached by the end of each circuit naturally leads to a deeper FIT recovery period, lasting about two to three minutes.

When you master two circuits, add a third, keeping the reps at 15, so long as you maintain perfect form throughout the entire circuit.

The target intensity index for this is Level 3. Think about it in terms of starting at a Salutation set level and gradually moving up to an Engagement set level. Even with the lightest starting weight, you will find your intensity reaching the Level 4 range at the end of each circuit.

You can do this workout at home—even without dumbbells. Use body-weight-only exercises such as those in the Base Camp sequence.

FIT Stretch

After your strength circuit you enjoy a series of six stretches. Stretching improves the range of motion of your joints, increases flexibility of your connective tissues and muscles, alleviates stress, and helps you stay injury-free. It's important that you hold the stretches, breathing deeply (as in your FIT recovery breathing—belly-style) as you deepen the stretch. Each stretch is held for 30 seconds, your initial target. Over the course of the TTC, increase the duration of each stretch until you reach a target of 60 seconds.

Be sure not to bounce on your stretches; hold them firm and steady, seeking to deepen gradually as you exhale. Stretching is an intelligent way to embrace your full body, helping you recover from this week's training.

Sunday: The 7th Day Away

Your body and mind require rest, recovery, and, as we discussed in Chapter 10, more calories. That's why every week during your Transformation you must take a day away from your training. Similar to the 7th day away in your Nutrition Plan, please don't get stuck in an overachieving mind-set, believing that doing more will somehow get you better results, faster. This is not the case. The opposite is true. Overtraining actually hinders your progress and sets you back.

Instead, enjoy this much needed mental and physical space from your training. Allow your body to build up and recuperate as your mind rejuvenates. This important 7th day away helps build your desire to reengage on Monday with renewed energy and strength.

Your Post-Workout 1-2-3

1. Record. Post your workout stats. Record your sets, reps, and intensity.

2. Project. Look forward and plan your next workout. Use this moment of clarity to establish your sets, reps, and weight that you will be using next time.

3. Reflect. Review the workout from your subjective view, inner thoughts. Journal.

Track and *Record* your accomplishments at the completion of each set. As part of your Recovery phase, quickly write down the number of completed reps, weight, and intensity.

At the end of your workout take advantage of your fresh clarity and *Project* forward: Write in your target weight for each set and exercise for the same day next week. Note areas where your intensity could have been higher, if you had too many and/or too few reps, and plan next week's workout accordingly. For example, at the close of the Push workout, plan next Monday's training session based on how you performed in the workout just completed. When next Monday rolls around, you will be properly prepared for the workout ahead without the hassle of trying to recall last week's accomplishments and adjusting on the fly.

When you plan in advance, you are more focused during training. You have clarity, and thus all your effort is reserved for the attainment of your plan. Treat your workout like it's a single event—one tennis match—rather than separate parts, making it a seamless integration from start to finish. Remember, if you don't know where you're going, you'll never get there! Know your plan, get in, check the clock, work out, and get out.

Finally, *Reflect* on your experience and success. This is where you write down a few high points and insights from your workout. This includes whatever you feel is most important—if something limited your success, like "didn't get enough sleep last night," note it. You'll be surprised how this helps you learn and evolve your training.

Use the bottom section of the Tracking Form. As you progress, and for months or more afterward, you'll find these notes along your path to be priceless.

ADD STRENGTH: STRATEGIES TO IMPROVE YOUR STRENGTH AND TRAINING

It is my wish that you not just "get through" your Transformation, but embrace training as an integral part of your life. And there's no question that we are inclined to embrace activities in which we have some degree of aptitude. We take joy in our skills and getting better, and the following strategies are ways to get better—to take you beyond the ordinary to the highly skilled.

These are not the essentials, but insider knowledge that can take an already sound practice deeper, to go beyond the basics and build a practice of *Strength for Life*.

Whether a good reminder or an epiphany, these strategies warrant your attention now and even more so later. Read them and come back to them often. At the end of your first month take a fresh look at these strategies. Each time you come back you will find a new depth, richness, and texture to apply to your training.

RITUAL OF PREPARATION

The focused performer is present in the moment. She's centered, mind free from random thoughts or irrelevant conversations. She doesn't use her training time for small talk or business conversation. Instead, she's totally focused on the task at hand.

Can you imagine what it would be like if you could apply this single-minded, laserlike focus and energy to all aspects of your life? Too often we become distracted and allow ourselves to think that "multitasking" is productive. In reality, we seem busy, but we're not accomplishing much of anything.

For as long as I can remember, I've had a ritual leading up to my training. On my way to train I like to clear my head from the day's activities. That means turning off the cell phone, shifting my focus from work, and putting on some tunes to get me in my training zone. Perhaps you've seen athletes perform a ritual in a pregame warm-up. A pretraining ritual works for me, and I believe it can help set the tone for your training too. You'll show up stronger, more focused, and ready to go.

Your ability to focus through strength training is a metaphor for the rest of your life. If you can't focus in the gym, your results will be modest—not insignificant, but only a fraction of what you could achieve. The same is true with life. Through FIT, you can learn to focus in your training, and that will translate into all aspects of your life.

BEST TIME TO TRAIN

Morning or later in the day? There are some advantages to training for each. Neither option will either make or break you. What will break you: missing your workout or being inconsistent. So the best time of day to train is the time that works best for you, day in, day out. That's a nice way of saying there is no perfect time—it's personal.

Pick a training time and stick to it.

AT HOME OR THE GYM

I designed the TTC around the use of dumbbells, which makes it possible to train at home, a convenient choice for many. All you need is a basic set of dumbbells and a bench. My choice for a home dumbbell set is PowerBlocks—an ingenious, space-saving invention. In just a few square feet you can have an instant, at-home Transformation center.

I train at home most of the time but truly enjoy and appreciate great gyms with a positive environment. There are tremendous advantages to training at a gym, be it a locally owned health club, city recreation center, or one of the national or global fitness chains. These gyms typically offer several ways in which to work your body with machines, dumbbells, and cardio equipment, as well as the space to stretch and train your core.

Another benefit of training in the gym is the availability of qualified trainers to help coach, inspire, and instruct you on proper form, provide valuable spotting techniques, and keep you on track to reach your goals. For many, health clubs also offer a social environment members both enjoy and depend on to stay the course.

If you should choose to train at a fitness center or gym, as many do, in Appendix F you will find a guide showing you corresponding gym equivalent exercise options.

Home or at the gym, the choice is yours.

TRAIN STRONG NOT LONG

A fundamental principle I've espoused for years is you can train long or train with intensity, but not both. Effective training is not necessarily tied to the duration of your workout but the intensity with which you approach each exercise throughout the week. Your TTC looks like this:

- Monday, Wednesday, and Thursday strength training workouts last approximately 33 to 44 minutes.
- Tuesday and Thursday cardio workouts last for 20 minutes, followed by another 12 to 15 minutes of abs.
- Saturday full-body FIT lasts for 20 minutes, followed by about 8 to 12 minutes of stretching.

The duration varies depending upon where you are in the Transformation cycle.

BE CAUSE, NOT EFFECT

There are two distinct ways of approaching the weights that make for remarkably different results: cause and effect.

Most people allow the weights to define their workout. They lift the dumbbell first, allowing their bodies to react. In essence, they're *in effect* of the weight. Weights create resistance, which in turn generates intensity in the muscles, causing the mind to briefly focus before the set is ended:

Focus ← Intensity ← Weight

This is a common approach to training. Most people, not knowing it can be different, unwittingly train this way every day. As you might guess, it's not the most effective, rewarding, or enjoyable way to train.

The other way (yes, there is another way), which you'll be doing with FIT, is one of those seemingly subtle shifts that can literally change everything—it will help you get more out of every rep and set than nearly anyone else in the gym.

When applying FIT, you are present, centered, and focused *prior* to even touching the weights. As you pick up the weight to begin your set, your focus immediately generates intensity, which *then* moves the weight. You feel the power of controlling the weight with your strength. This is training *at cause*:

Focus → Intensity → Weight

When you use your focus to generate the highest levels of intensity, the degree of muscular engagement is exponentially greater than if you wait for the weights to trigger the intensity. You're more in tune with your training, enjoying an experience that yields greater results.

LESS WEIGHT, MORE STRENGTH

As important as mental focus and physical intensity are to results, form—good technique in your training—is not optional. Bring the most focused mind and strong body to training with sloppy form, and you've got, at best, a waste of time, and at worst, injury.

Too often form is sacrificed in the name of lifting more weight. In the TTC you integrate the FIT sequence into your training, making it an ideal time to also lower the amount of weight you typically use, to emphasize near perfect form on every set.

As you develop your focus and intensity through FIT, you will be making ever greater gains with less weight, so take this time to focus on your form and technique. Don't make the amount of weight your central focus. Use less weight in your training and bring more strength of body and mind.

PICK THE RIGHT STARTING WEIGHT

If you have no idea of your strength levels, finding the right weight to begin is simple trial and error. It's a process of becoming familiar with your strength. Remember, *focus* and *form* come first—weight is an asset to be leveraged, not something to organize around to the exclusion of all else.

My advice is to start light and develop your comfort, confidence, and coordination before beginning the gradual progression up in weight for each of your TTC sets.

ADJUSTING YOUR WEIGHTS

For the 12-rep Salutation set, choose a weight that, if needed, you can do about 20 to 25 times. For the 10-rep Engagement set, use a weight you can actually complete about 15 times. And for the Activation and Challenge sets you want a weight you can perform 8 times.

The rules for adjusting up—and in some cases down—are simple. On your final 8-rep upper-body Challenge set, if you fail to complete 6 full reps, decrease the weight by five pounds. If you get more than 10 reps, increase your weight by five pounds for your next workout. For a 10-rep Challenge set, the rules are the same. It's plus or minus 2 reps. This means if you're between 8 and 12, stay at the same weight. If you drop below 8 reps, lower the weight. If you hit a baker's dozen, increase the weight.

For lower-body exercises, use these same guidelines to increase or decrease the weight; however, instead of making changes in five-pound increments, make adjustments in ten-pound increments for your next workout.

Quick Guide:

- **Number of reps are less than 6, adjust down 5 pounds (10 for legs)**
- **Number of reps are between 6 and 10, stay at this weight**
- **Number of reps are greater than 10, go up 5 pounds (10 for legs)**

BE PROGRESSIVE

The human body is incredibly adaptive, constantly reaching for a balance between its capacities and demands. The body never stands still, it either gets stronger or weaker. By pushing your upper limits in both your strength and cardio training, you ask your body to expand its capacities.

The TTC is a *progressive* program. That is, it consistently increases the demands on your body over time.

Progression sparks the improvements you make over the course of your Transformation, be it increasing the weight you can lift or the number of reps you can achieve with a given weight. You may see it in the increased cardio intensity as your intervals reach higher peaks.

WHAT GOES UP, MUST COME DOWN

In any complete strength training movement there are two distinct phases: the *concentric* phase, when you lift the weight up; and the *eccentric* phase, when you lower the weight. Each phase is performed with an equal amount of concentration and effort. Good lifting is a controlled art form focusing on both movements equally.

One of the greatest errors people make in strength training is focusing only on the concentric phase of the lift—the pressing, pushing, or pulling. If you fail to control the weight throughout the entire lift, you are only getting half of the benefit. Stay in complete command of the weight on the way up *and* down. The eccentric portion of the lift has been shown to increase strength at a faster rate than training concentric contractions alone.

This whole process, raising and lowering the weight, is seamless and fluid.

MAKE EVERY REP COUNT

I have found that people often focus on the total rep target (12, 10, 8, etc.). They make it a race to get the final rep, but their in-between reps suffer. This is where your mind–muscle link needs to come in. Learn to maximize it by treating every rep of every set as if it's the only one that counts. When you're pushing with all your force for one rep, it forces you to summon your intensity.

Counting strong can help you stay focused, getting the most from each rep. Count both movements, the concentric and eccentric, in each rep. During the up movement you always silently count "One" for each rep in the set. On the way down you count the number of reps you have completed during the set so far. Putting it together looks like this:

Rep 1: On the way up, "One." On the way down, "One."
Rep 2: On the way up, "One." On the way down, "Two."
Rep 3: On the way up, "One." On the way down, "Three."

And so forth.

Sounds simple, but there's a subtle power in this. Your attention is not on the destination—but on the quality of each rep, in the moment.

If you're just starting out, you may want to count the rep you're completing twice on the way down to help you master your lifting cadence. For example:

Rep 1: On the way up, "One." On the way down, "One, one."

Rep 2: On the way up, "One." On the way down, "Two, two."

Rep 3: On the way up, "One." On the way down, "Three, three."

TOUCH TRAINING

Just as it sounds, touch training means touching the active muscle during the exercise. It's an effective way to increase Peak Intensity.

Touching the muscle you're training focuses your mind on that point, igniting the connection between your mind and the muscle. Not only does this technique work in practice, science has also demonstrated that touch can increase the neurological activation between the mind and body to strengthen the ability to contract the muscle.

Touch training has been practiced for decades, and once you use it, you'll know why. It works and it's simple to do. For an example of touch training in action, recall the exercise from Chapter 3 with the biceps curl.

REFLECTIONS OF STRENGTH

Have you ever wondered why gym walls are covered with mirrors? So people can look at themselves, of course. Actually, there's another more valuable reason.

As you know, the quality of any exercise depends upon the degree of focus. Focus is powerfully influenced by your vision, because the eyes deliver information rapidly to the brain. Mirrors provide a full view of your body and your muscles, helping you to improve mental focus as well as maintain good form. You literally focus on what you see.

Simply looking at a muscle can make an immediate difference. Just try it. While curling a dumbbell, close your eyes or look at the ceiling—look anywhere but at your biceps. Maintaining the mental focus on your biceps is a huge challenge.

Now feel the difference by curling the same weight, with the same arm, but remaining intensely focused on the biceps. Watch it move, see it, and *feel* it with your eyes. The difference is significant.

Your back is a unique and special case in training for it's always there, right behind you—and as such, you can't see it in the mirror. As a result of this visual disconnect, many people either skip over back training or fail to train their back effectively. It helps to have a mirror that allows you to see a side view of yourself while training, but the trick to back training is to visualize and connect with your back muscles through your mind's eye. Perfect this skill in your back training and you'll improve in every lift—with every muscle.

BREATHE IN THE AIR

Breathing is vital to successful strength training. Unfortunately, many make this natural activity a hindrance, either breathing incorrectly or even holding their breath during training. Holding your breath is counterproductive, if not altogether dangerous.

Proper breathing boosts focus and intensity when done in a simple, consistent pattern in rhythm with your movements. While lowering the weight (eccentric phase), inhale, breathing into your lungs. While lifting the weight (concentric phase), exhale. This applies to all strength training exercises.

Your breath acts as a focal point for your mind in each exercise. Placing your attention on your breathing is the gateway for your mind to become in sync with your body and the movements of each repetition.

As you advance in your FIT practice, breathing becomes an integrated, fluid expression of your focus and intensity, allowing you to then place your awareness on proper form and immediate sensations within the muscles you're training.

ADAPTATION PERIOD

If you're new to lifting weights or are just getting "back at it" after an extended layoff, the first four to six weeks will be spent developing your neurological system—the wiring between your mind and muscles. This necessary step precedes the increase in lean, shape-defining muscle.

First, you must be able to activate and engage the muscle *you already* have. As your nervous system develops, you will experience significant gains in strength. Much like the ability to ride a bike, which requires intense concentration at first, your training coordination and skill improve as you develop this "wiring"—equipping you for a lifetime of strength.

MUSCLE SORENESS

Intense strength training will result in muscle soreness, typically a day or two following your workout. If you're not accustomed to awakening your body's strength in this fashion, it's helpful to interpret these sensations more accurately as signs of success. That's right—your muscles are telling you that you have successfully challenged them and they are at this moment improving to meet your request. It's a wonderful positive sign.

After two or three weeks of consistent training, muscle soreness will significantly dissipate. As long as you train regularly, it will become nothing more than a subtle sense of having trained a muscle—nothing dramatic but rather a good feeling.

FOLLOW YOUR HEART

The Focus Intensity Index provides a reliable way for gauging and tracking your intensity during your strength training. But how do you know where you're at, intensity-wise, on cardio?

In the interest of keeping the low end low and the high end high, I've added a heart-rate monitor to my list of essential training gear. When I'm doing any cardio, I train with a heart-rate monitor, and highly recommend that you get one too.

When it comes to cardio, heart-rate monitors are one of the best tools for monitoring your training performance and improvement. I regularly maintain about a 20 percent higher output when my heart-rate monitor is in place and giving me live feedback. It keeps me where I want to be, getting the most out of every minute. Follow the guidelines for your age as provided by your professional trainer and/or the literature that comes with a quality heart-rate monitor.

FEEL YOUR STRENGTH

Remember, the only things worth having are those for which you have to work. The demand you place on yourself will only be exceeded by the rewards you receive. Your view of your own abilities will change upon the completion of this program. Train hard, stay dedicated, eat right, and get plenty of sleep, and this program will be the most productive cycle of training you have ever enjoyed.

Week 13 and Beyond: 12 Months That Will Set You Free

Good actions give strength to ourselves and inspire good actions in others.
—PLATO

CHAPTER 12

Beyond the Transformation

Congratulations on your accomplishments! You've made it to the finish line—you are success-fully through your Transformation.

In the opening pages of this book I invited you to create a turning point in your life. In Chapter 1, I challenged you to go beyond health and adopt strength as your guiding value, ac-cepting nothing less than a life of abundant energy and vitality. You are now part of an elite group who, with strength as a guiding value, have mobilized the focus, heart, and courage to make this leap.

As you recall, the *Strength for Life* program has three distinct phases: start strong, get strong, and stay strong. You started strong in the 12 days of Base Camp and excelled in the 12-week TTC to get strong, testing your inner strength and forging your outer. You've learned a lot about yourself—it's been a transformative few months. You've taken a step toward your full potential.

Now it's time to step *beyond* your Transformation to discover how to stay strong: for the next 12 months and for life. The annual plan you create will have you reaching new levels of fitness year after year, keeping you motivated, inspired, and going strong.

You now have the honor of greeting a new challenge—one known only to the finishers like you—the challenge of balancing the quest for continued progress with a sustainable fitness lifestyle. Benefiting from the lessons of those who have come before, in this chapter I'll show you how to integrate what you've learned in the TTC, while avoiding the pitfalls that can de-rail you.

LESSONS FROM WEEK 13 AND BEYOND: MISTAKES YOU WON'T MAKE

One of the challenges that many have faced and struggled with is precisely where you are now. You may be asking, "What comes after the Transformation?" This seemingly innocent Week 13 has been the beginning of the end for many in years past.

At the end of a Transformation, people commonly make the mistake of continuing on as if the finish line has moved. Enthused by visible results, they seek ever greater progress, one intense week after another. Others recognize the end of the 12 weeks and dutifully begin back at Week 1 all over again. Either way, this quest for constant improvement zaps your motivation and drains you physically and mentally. Eventually, overcome by fatigue, you can no longer continue.

While forging on with a Transformation beyond Week 12 shows heart and desire, it is neither wise nor optimal. In their enthusiasm for ever-greater results, these people fail to recognize that a Transformation is an intensive 12-week phase of conditioning designed specifically to *transform,* not as a sustainable lifestyle.

Going through the intense rigors of back-to-back Transformations with no pause for recovery is the equivalent of an athlete enduring back-to-back seasons without a break. It's simply too much. Absent the necessary downtime for complete and full recovery, the very things that trigger your body to become leaner and stronger will quickly start working against you. As a result, your body begins to break down muscle, dissolving all your hard-won achievements.

If you are thinking, "Not me, I have done back-to-back Transformations," I can assure you that you did not push yourself to your limits during your Transformation. If you're feeling as if you could stick with the Transformation Training indefinitely, you've most likely allowed your training intensity to drop to a maintenance level. The sure sign that you've been bringing your full concentrated "Level 5" intensity is that by Week 12 you'll be *ready* to turn down the heat. Similar to the peak intervals in your HIIT: If you don't have to resist turning down the intensity, you're *not* at your limits and not maximizing your results.

Still others choose to cease training altogether after a Transformation. Acting as if they've reached the end of a race, they stop running, sit down, and promptly forget everything they've learned. Their training declines and their nutrition suffers as they revert to their life as it was before Transformation. I can assure you this is *not* what you want to do.

When it comes to *Week 13 and beyond,* the successes and failures of those who have gone before serve as our guideposts. From them we learn what works and what does not. We can see that should we hold on too tightly, continuing to pursue ever greater improvements without recovery, we actually may set ourselves back. If we fail to embrace what we learned from the Transformation, we are destined to drift helplessly back to mediocrity.

Why have so many struggled to sustain their gains—let alone improve—following a Transformation? The answer is simple: They were left to find their own way. That's not going to happen to you. Rather than becoming another dropout statistic, burnt out from repeated Transformations, I've got another plan for you.

BUILDING YOUR MUSCLE OF APPRECIATION

There's no question that the lack of guidance for Week 13 and beyond has contributed to people attempting to make a Transformation a year-round event, but it's by no means the only factor. Certainly much of the blame must go to society's insatiable thirst for *more*—more money, more time, more freedom, more food . . . more everything. We've made quantity king and quality the rare exception.

We're always looking toward the horizon—to our next attainment. We're never satisfied. And how can we be when we so rarely take the time to strengthen our muscle of appreciation? When it comes to accomplishments such as completing a Transformation, we're quick to express frustration with lack of progress, yet we tend not to credit ourselves enough, if at all.

This phenomenon can even be seen in many who enjoy astounding Transformation success. They've made what looks to be a year's progress in mere weeks but are so preoccupied with getting better, being leaner and more fit, that they fail to recognize just how far they've come.

Recognize these people with a comment, "You look great!" and you may receive a response like, "Well, I'm working on a few things . . . could be better."

Their new, improved self has become their new baseline—each step up is a new "square one" starting point. For them to be happy again, they must "take it up" one more level. It's no mystery why they eventually run out of steam. Rather than appreciating their progress and allowing their bodies and minds to recharge, they start *again,* which is really *to continue.* They return to Week 1, but their body is saying "unlucky Week 13" loud and clear.

Whether you have met or surpassed your highest goals or missed it by a few inches or pounds, your achievements are significant. If you choose to measure your success only by the scale, the tape, or even your eye, as many do, you're missing more than half the picture. Your true measure of success resides much deeper. The full magnitude of your results can be found *and* felt inside—in your energy, confidence, and strength.

For whatever the distance to your ultimate Vision, it's time to stop looking to the horizon, pursuing perfection. This is the moment to celebrate your success. I'm inviting you, without an option of decline, to recognize your achievements and appreciate what you've accomplished over the past 12 weeks.

If, like most of us, you are uncertain how to do this, the following brief exercise will help you reflect and gain perspective on what you've learned, the skills you've gained, the obstacles you've overcome, and the strength you've embodied through your Transformation. This three-step exercise takes less than ten minutes. Here's what I'd like you to do:

Step one: Grab a blank sheet of paper and a pen. Then set a timer for five minutes (a watch, clock, cell phone, anything that can track time works).

Step two: Start your timer and begin writing down all the positives, the many successes you have experienced during the last 12 weeks of the TTC. Let them flow to your mind unedited—if it comes up, big or small, write it down. Even something as seemingly insignificant as, "I didn't eat any mayonnaise on a sandwich," write it down. And keep writing until your five minutes are up.

Ready, set, go! Do this now. You can return to read the final step when you're done filling the page with positives.

Step three: You're done. Now take a two-minute break. When back from your break, I want you to read each item you wrote on that paper, *aloud*. Read them as if you're telling someone you care deeply about. As you complete each item, allow yourself to feel the gratitude and respect.

I have found this exercise to be a vital step in redirecting the natural tendency to focus on the slips or miscues, as most of us have been conditioned to focus on what we don't want. By calling your focus to all you've done right, you further fuel your success and motivation. As always, success begets success. Giving yourself totally to a goal for a set period of time is literally molding, shaping, and forging your will. You should be proud of your achievement, as I know you are.

Upon realizing Transformation success, I've found people are inclined to give credit elsewhere: to the program, a book, or even its author. This achievement is all yours. The completion of your Transformation is an expression of your resolve and a testament to your inner strength. After all, you brought the focus and intensity to your training, you changed the way you enjoyed food, and you courageously reshaped your destiny. Truly it is you who have done the noble work.

If you created an incentive in advance of your Transformation—a reward for your completion—terrific. This is the time to deliver on your self-promise. It may be a vacation, a special dinner, a day off of work, or a round of golf. Whatever it is, go now and enjoy.

If you didn't plan an incentive for yourself, you can still come up with something special now. No need to go overboard, but go ahead and give yourself a tangible reward. What's most important is that you stop, recognize, and honor *your* effort and commitment.

As you reflect on your Transformation, you may find yourself changed in ways you never considered. People often begin a Transformation motivated by a prize, money, or even the thrill of competition, but when they come through, it's the satisfaction, increased confidence, and freedom that is the real prize. Almost universally, every person who's successfully completed a Transformation that I've spoken with has commented on this welcome yet unexpected shift.

TAKE SEVEN

In Chapters 6 and 7 you set a compelling vision and Transformation goals, and in the previous exercise you made peace with your goals and recognized your successes. Regardless of how accurately you aimed and hit, once you've reached the close of the TTC, the buzzer sounds. Time's up! That's it. Do not allow yourself to squeeze out another week or even one more day. It's time to recharge and reflect.

In recognition of your hard-earned accomplishments, and serving your best interests, my gift to you is Week 13: take 7 days away. The only thing I want you to do now is nothing! That's right, not a single thing. No strength training, no cardio training, make it one long 7th day away, if you like. Respect yourself, your recovery, and the wisdom I'm offering—give yourself a break.

You can eat, however, whenever you like. Although my guess is you won't veer too far off course, as once you reexperience what lousy food does to your body and how it tanks your energy, especially in excess, you'll go with the good feeling and come right back to eating well.

This week off is a powerful experience for many people who fear that time away from training or even one meal will cost them their hard-earned gains. Some resist relaxing even for a moment in fear they will lose it all. You must be able to relax your grip, for it's invariably those who try the hardest never to slip up, allowing themselves no room for error, who eventually unravel. They tend to go from eating like a saint to dining with the devil.

If this full week free causes you unrest, relax. It's seven short days and you need and deserve it. You will return revived, rested, and ready to embrace a sustainable annual plan for your strength, fitness, and freedom.

In the rest of Section 4 we'll fill in the final piece to your *Strength for Life* plan. In the next chapter I'll show you how to generate a sustainable path with a rhythm and pace that fits your life and your natural training style—the right way forward for you. In Chapter 14 we'll look directly into and behind *the mechanics of motivation* to discover how you can evolve your motivation for a lifetime of strength and fitness mastery. You do that which you are motivated to do. And by *doing,* there comes a point where staying strong and fit is no longer *what you do* but becomes *who you are.* How do you become one of those rare few whose zeal for living grows with each passing year—who continues to improve? In Chapter 15 we look into the lives of the group with the most to teach us—the Transformed. Those who didn't just change their body and snap a photo, but were truly Transformed, from the inside out, providing great insight to sustaining your *best for life.*

For now, kick back, relax, and enjoy.

CHAPTER 13

Seasons of Strength

One of my favorite sporting events of the year is the pinnacle of bike racing—the Tour de France. Several years ago, up before the early July sun, I found myself enthralled in the live television coverage as Lance Armstrong continued his domination on the way to winning his record breaking seventh Tour. Lance's dedication to this one cycling event each year is legendary. He trained exclusively to win the race that defines cycling, accepting nothing less than his absolute best. The results of his focus on this one peak performance per year speak for themselves.

As I watched Lance pull away on a hill climb, I had an epiphany: The clarity and focus of this annual peaking *ritual* was actually the secret to sustaining fitness for life. The answer to the question of how you stay strong and fit for life had become clear. You don't. Instead, you get in your absolute best shape once a year, year after year. The key to staying in shape for life is giving your life shape: clearly defined, meaningful peaks when you aim beyond your best. It's in pushing the bounds of the possible that you expand your limits.

If you recall from Chapter 2, The Shape of Your Life, the Transformation Training Camp is a finely tuned peak phase for transforming your body. It works like a booster rocket, breaking you free from the gravity of health and elevating you toward a life of strength. Like all training camps, it comes to an end. Athletes don't spend 365 days a year in their peak physical condition; instead, they organize their lives and performance around seasons. They know when to peak, when to maintain, and when to recharge their bodies and minds.

The Tour de France provided a rhythm, focus, and motivating deadline to Lance's training. Just as the Tour was his single organizing event of the year, I want you to think of the TTC as *your* organizing event—your peak season. The TTC provides rhythm, focus, and structure to your 12-month plan that has you reaching new levels of *strength and fitness* each year—while fueling your off-peak training. The new challenges that each season brings inspire renewed energy and commitment, keeping you fresh and focused.

The logic is sound: Get in your best shape one time each year and you'll be in shape for life.

Your season of strength (the TTC) culminates in your *Peak Performance Day*—the day in which you complete your Transformation—when you're in the best shape of the year. Your fitness calendar is organized around this day. For your *next* Transformation, you'll choose a peak date that works best for you. You may end your Transformation just prior to your annual vacation, taking time off while feeling and looking great. You'll also get to enjoy the benefit of making the vacation a reward for your efforts. Or set your peak date for your birthday or prior to summer so you're in top shape to enjoy your favorite outdoor activities.

Once you've chosen your Peak Performance Day, count backward 14 weeks to start your Transformation. Why 14? Because for each Transformation you'll invest 12 days in Base Camp prior to entering your 12-week climb. That leaves you with about three 12-week seasons remaining in the year. These are your off-peak training seasons. Your off-peak training is oriented around sustainability and is not to be confused with time off (i.e., seven days away). In your off-peak training—before and after your Transformations—you can spend more time on a favorite form of exercise such as yoga, aerobics, or kung-fu. You name it.

When you embarked on your Transformation, you did so with a history—a fitness history, that is. Were you running, swimming, or cycling? Competing in triathlons? Perhaps you already had a steady practice of weight training. Do you enjoy stretching your limits with yoga or the precision and challenge of martial arts? Maybe you've done nothing for years.

We all have different strengths, talents, skills, and fitness styles. In my case it's clear, I'm not a runner. A sprinter, yes. A runner, no. I find running unbelievably painful on multiple levels. In my formative years I excelled at sports that involved power and short bursts of strength. I played football, wrestled, and sprinted in track. Sprinterlike bursts of strength are in my DNA. That's my fitness style. What's yours? If you don't know immediately, think back. Your history shines light on your exercise preference—*your* natural fitness style.

As you know by now, strength training is important for a lifetime of freedom, strength, and energy. However, it is *not* my intention to overwrite your natural fitness style. You do not have to lift weights three times a week all year long to stay strong and fit, but by integrating strength training into your annual plan, you'll be on the path to a lifetime of strength and fitness.

THE CORNERSTONES OF FITNESS

Strength, Stamina, and *Stretch* (*Flexibility*) are the three Cornerstones of Fitness from which you'll build your annual plan. While nearly any sport, exercise, or activity involves all three of these dimensions in differing degrees, each has its primary or leading emphasis. For instance, it takes strength to run a marathon, but it's easy to see that it's primarily an event of extraordinary endurance or stamina.

The three cornerstones defined are:

Strength: The realm of developing strong sculpted muscles, primarily through strength training or other forms of resistance training. It's the leading dimension of the Transformation you just completed. Strength, ultimately, is your physical and mental power.

Stamina: Refers to your cardiovascular endurance—your ability to exert physical and mental energy over long periods of time. This is primarily associated with distance running, cycling, and swimming; however, many other activities such as HIIT develop stamina.

Stretch (Flexibility): Stretching is the process of lengthening or extending the muscles, tendons, and ligaments, increasing your body's overall range of motion. It supports the suppleness of your joints and body in general. It's a capacity perhaps most refined in the yoga traditions.

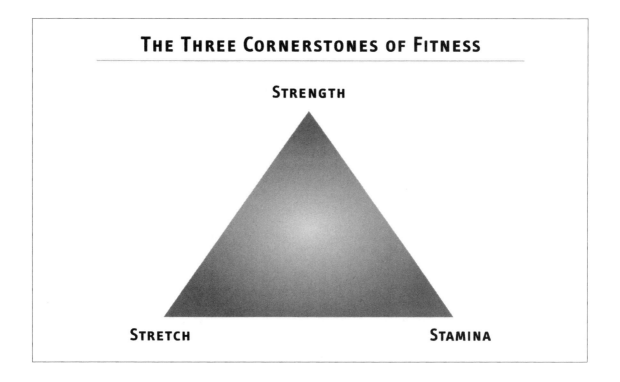

THE THREE CORNERSTONES OF FITNESS

STRENGTH

STRETCH

STAMINA

THE PERFECT IMBALANCE

Your Transformation training integrates each of the three Cornerstones of Fitness; not in balance, but rather, in perfect imbalance. The TTC is first and foremost Strength, with Stamina a strong second, and Flexibility in support. When it comes to defining the other seasons of your training year, whatever your fitness preference, you will apply a similar imbalance, leading with the cornerstone of your choice—the other two in service of this emphasis.

To improve in any dimension of fitness, be it Strength, Stamina, or Flexibility, you must lead with one dimension at a time, which is to choose imbalance. Training with the aim to simultaneously balance two or three dimensions of fitness is actually counterproductive. To be "out of balance" in your training is what creates real progress.

As I mentioned in Chapter 4, lean muscle and strength are best cultivated while minimizing endurance training. Both Strength and Stamina are vital elements of fitness, but are competing dimensions and cannot be optimally trained at the same time. Competing commitments divert your energy and focus, resulting in nominal improvements at best, and in many cases prove to be extremely inefficient and terribly frustrating. Aim for perfect balance and you'll find yourself putting in much higher effort with less return.

The idea that one could possess heroic strength, gymnastlike flexibility, and inexhaustible stamina at the same time makes for a great comic book character. But even superheroes know that to actually "be super" they must possess specialized focus and talent.

SHAPING YOUR SEASONS WITH FORMULA 4:2:1

Formula 4:2:1 is a guide for defining your seasons of training in concert with the Cornerstones of Fitness. Each cornerstone is assigned a value in order of its primary emphasis for the season. Your lead Cornerstone is assigned a 4, your supporting cornerstones are assigned 2 and 1, respectively. Each number represents a combination of time *and* intensity of training—or what you might best call *total effort.*

It's a half-half ratio: halve 4 and you get 2; halve 2 and you get 1. Spend about half the amount of time that you train in your lead cornerstone on your secondary dimension, halve that again and you have the approximate time to spend on the remaining cornerstone.

Put another way, in a clock world, for about every 40 minutes training your lead cornerstone, you spend 20 and 10 minutes respectively in your supporting dimensions. For example, let's say you apply your 4:2:1 to a season of stretch, stamina, and strength, in that order. In any given week you allocate three hours to a relatively challenging style of yoga (Lead Cornerstone:

Flexibility), 90 minutes training your stamina (Secondary Cornerstone), followed by 45 minutes of strength training (Support Cornerstone). In this scenario you'll spend a little over five hours total training for the week. This may be split up over five days, or perhaps some days you'll stack your training by hitting two dimensions in the same day. Here's a look at how you might accomplish this in four days:

7-DAY OFF-PEAK: FLEXIBILITY LEAD

MON	TUES	WED	THURS	FRI	SAT	SUN
STAMINA STRETCH 30 MINUTES CARDIO 1 HOUR YOGA	OFF	**STRETCH** 1 HOUR YOGA ABS	OFF	**STRETCH** 1 HOUR YOGA ABS	**FULL BODY** 45 MINUTES FIT CIRCUIT 30 MINUTES CARDIO	OFF

As you know, your total effort and intensity impacts the quality of your training, so use your time wisely.

Formula 4:2:1 is your perfect imbalance that helps ensure that you focus in one area for a season while sustaining progress in the other areas, with no one dimension ignored during any training week. It's worth emphasizing that the numbers are meant as a guide, *not* an absolute. For example, the TTC is a 4:2:1 of Strength-Stamina-Stretch, though it's actually a bit heavy on strength due to the emphasis on shaping your body. Additionally, the TTC highly values training intensity over duration.

Now, there's always exceptions to the rule. If you're training for a sport or competitive event, you either have a coach or know how to get the information you need to train accordingly. For example, a distance runner spends considerable time developing stamina, beyond the 4:2:1 ratio, as does the person embarking on a competitive season in any sport. Similarly, if you're a fifth-degree black belt or Cirque de Soleil performer able to do a one-finger handstand, you may have strength mastered and require a different training emphasis. Likewise, yoga masters who possess amazing strength and flexibility may desire a unique ratio that embraces their practice. If you're one of these exceptions, you know who you are. Use good judgment and remember: Formula 4:2:1 requires that you spend at least some time training in each dimension during your week. It supports clear focal points and enhances a lifetime of sustainability. It's the variety and structure that keep you steadily evolving in an integrated way.

FORMULA 4:2:1 AT WORK

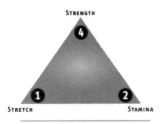

TTC Peak Season
Strength 4: Stamina 2: Stretch 1

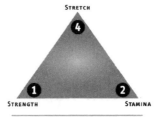

Off-Peak Season Example 1
Stretch 4: Stamina 2: Strength 1

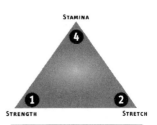

Off-Peak Season Example 2
Stamina 4: Stretch 2: Strength 1

Formula 4:2:1 is a half-half ratio. Halve 4 and you get 2; halve 2 and you get 1. Spend about half the time you train in your lead cornerstone on your secondary cornerstone, halve that again for the time to train on your remaining cornerstone. Total effort and intensity impacts the quality of your training.

Nutrition: Keep Your Structure, Enjoy Your Freedom

Consuming nutritious, balanced meals five times daily, seven days a week is no small accomplishment. Maintaining it every day, 365 days, with hectic schedules, travel, and temptations is nothing short of heroic. The reality is, everyone—and this includes you—will at some point eat something other than an ideal, well-balanced meal.

Perhaps it will be a conscious choice to indulge or a moment of weakness brought on by hunger that leads you to a fast-food burger and fries or some sugar-filled treat. Whatever the case, just realize that this is not the end of the world. Slip-ups happen—that's a given. Where it becomes an issue of concern is when a slip turns into a slide and you go off the deep end, jamming down a half-dozen doughnuts and abandoning your positive relationship with food.

Accounting for the constant pursuit of perfection in our culture, you may find the "80 percent rule" to be a valuable ally for supporting your Nutritional Freedom in off-peak seasons. What this means is, if you eat the right foods at the right times in the right amounts about 80 percent of the time (four out of five meals), you'll continue to maintain your Transformation results. Rather than letting a single imperfection in your eating trigger self-incrimination or some deep emotional flogging, just note it in your food journal, embrace it, and move on.

This strategy provides you with built-in wiggle room for eating so you can be less than perfect and still get back on track with your next meal. Remember, you're not dieting, but eating to live. To score 100 percent is your Transformation target, but when it comes to long-term results, practice your Nutritional Awareness and do the right thing 80 percent of the time.

General Parameters for Off-Peak Training

A season of training should be about 12 weeks, plus or minus a week. It depends on your annual plan and whether you choose to do one or two TTC phases each year. It's helpful to keep the training rhythm that you've set forth in your TTC. You've already learned to make the time, so keep the commitment.

General guidelines:

- Include all three cornerstones each week.
- You may enjoy between three and six training sessions each week. Most people find four or five to be the sweet spot.
- Allow yourself to experiment, leading with a new cornerstone at least one season a year. Let go of the idea that once you try something new, it's a lifetime commitment.
- Seek guidance from a trainer or other knowledgeable professional on proper form to improve your efficiency of movement and prevent injuries.

Training Your Cornerstone of Strength

In your off-peak training seasons, strength-train between one to four days per week. If you go with three days, you can adapt the TTC push/legs/pull regimen into a solid season by reducing the number of Focus Intensity Level 5 sets and drop sets. Keep your intensity levels in the three to four range with no more than one Level 5 per body part.

Multiple Transformations in the Same Year*

Perhaps you didn't attain all your goals in your Transformation and you're eager to return to the TTC right away. If you think you're ready, here's a sound, sensible approach to effectively manage two Transformations annually:

- No Transformations back-to-back.
- Take seven days away (you did this in Week 13).
- Go off-peak for one season (enjoy 12 weeks of training to your fitness style).
- Return to Base Camp for 12 days.
- Embark on your next TTC.

* If you insist, for a multitude of reasons, upon three Transformations annually, you must promise yourself to take at least four weeks of off-peak training in between each.

If you're looking for a way in which you can strength-train your entire body in two days, split your workouts into upper body and lower body. For one day of strength training you can use the Saturday Full-Body FIT while adding a third circuit so you have three full sets for each movement.

Variety has its place—it can freshen things up and challenge the body in new ways. A professional trainer can provide a program that fits into your season regardless of what leading cornerstone you've chosen.

Guidelines for your off-peak strength training:

- **Training sessions should last between 33 and 44 minutes.**
- **Maintain reps in the 10–15 range.**
- **Train each body part at least once each week.**
- **Do not work the same body parts two consecutive days.**
- **Use your knowledge from the TTC to enhance your training: Refer to Chapter 11 often.**

Just because you're practicing off-peak training does not mean you should not be making progress. You can and should continue to shape and refine your body, in whatever direction you choose. Use this time as an opportunity to strengthen and deepen your integration of body and mind with your FIT practice. Keep the pace of each rep *and* your training steady and smooth—not too fast but no slacking around. Don't build bad habits, but rather, improve your concentration and focus with practice. After your workout, remember Nutritional Freedom Strategy 8 and be sure to *Feed Your Strength* (see page 102).

Training Your Cornerstone of Stamina

When it comes to training your stamina in the off-peak seasons, there is no absolute formula. HIIT is still a terrific form of cardio. It's quick and effective, and you can maintain it if you've grown to prefer this form of stamina training.

If you're ready for a break from HIIT, you may choose to run on a treadmill, bike the hills, or even enjoy some swimming. It's your call. Go at it with all of your heart. Formula 4:2:1 keeps you from the common mistake so many make, training one dimension (stamina) in the absence of the others.

It's nice to change it up, and should you decide to, here are some basic guidelines for off-peak stamina training:

- **A non-HIIT stamina workout includes at least 30 minutes of maintaining a minimum target heart rate of 65 percent maximum.**
- **As you increase your stamina, begin to gradually increase the rate at which you're moving.**
- **Choose friendly surfaces to run on: tracks, grass, or sand. Dirt paths are excellent for variety and reducing joint stress. Avoid concrete and asphalt.**

- Remember to drink H$_2$O: Stay hydrated before, during, and after all workouts, especially stamina training.

Training Your Cornerstone of Stretch/Flexibility

The dimension of flexibility is quite likely the most overlooked of the three Cornerstones of Fitness. Why? Simply because most people don't think of the ability to touch their toes as a component of fitness. Thank goodness for yoga—for its impact has brought structure and consistency to stretching and opening the body and mind.

Should you be a devotee of yoga or some form of exercise that emphasizes the suppleness of the body, you will likely choose to lead a season with Stretch. I realize that my inclusion of yoga as a stretch practice may provoke response from some of the yoga persuasion. I include it here because it's my view that many people practice yoga largely to stretch and open the body. Yet clearly there are many derivations of yoga that have wide-reaching impact beyond flexibility, integrating strength, stamina, and body–mind connection.

A few basic guidelines for flexibility:

- Yoga sessions, in a season leading with Flexibility, are a minimum of 45 minutes.
- Stretch sessions, as supporting cornerstones, are a minimum of 15 minutes.
- You may include your flexibility as a conclusion to strength or stamina workouts.
- Slowly enter into and out of your stretches. Never bounce.
- Hold your stretches for 30 to 60 seconds.

If you choose to lead a season with Stretch, you may include three sessions of yoga in a week. As certain schools of yoga engage stamina and strength, you can stack multiple cornerstones in any given workout. But choose your yoga wisely so you don't make the common mistake of assuming this eliminates the need for training your support cornerstones.

PLANNING YOUR SEASONS OF STRENGTH: EASY AS 1-2-3

Step 1: Choose Your Peak Performance Day

Your annual strength and fitness plan begins by establishing your annual Peak Performance Day—your best shape of the year day. This is the day you complete your Transformation. When you establish this day, you create the momentum that shapes your entire year.

Write it in your calendar now.

Step 2: Determine Your Fitness Preference

Choose your fitness preference. It may be immediately apparent to you or an absolute mystery. If you don't know, reflect on your TTC and select your favorite dimension.

My natural fitness style is: _____

SEASONS OF STRENGTH

EXAMPLE	SEASON #1	SEASON #2	SEASON #3 TTC	SEASON #4
4	STAMINA	STRETCH	STRENGTH	STRENGTH
2	STRENGTH	STRENGTH	STAMINA	STRETCH
1	STRETCH	STAMINA	STRETCH	STAMINA

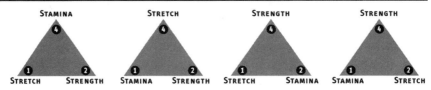

YOUR TURN	SEASON #1	SEASON #2	SEASON #3	SEASON #4
4				
2				
1				

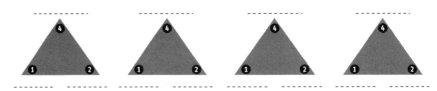

(Write in the appropriate cornerstone for each season on the lines provided)

Step 3: Define Your Training Seasons for the Year Ahead

Using your Peak Performance Day as the organizing point, the stake in the ground, divide the year ahead into four seasons. Next, select your lead and supporting cornerstones for each season. For your first off-peak season use your fitness preference as your leading style. I encourage you to switch your leading cornerstone for at least one season each year to embrace a new practice, push your limits. Or, if you wish, stick with the TTC schedule for an off-peak training season.

Now write in your Formula 4:2:1 for the next four seasons, one of which will be a Transformation. This calendar is dynamic, changing every Peak Performance Day.

STAY STRONG WITH AN ANNUAL PEAK PERFORMANCE DAY RITUAL

We don't all have a Tour de France to inspire us to be in our best shape every year. But you can create an inspiring annual ritual that will keep you on track.

In conjunction with your annual Peak Performance Day, get a complete physical checkup. Have all your vital stats checked. Check outside by taking an annual set of "after" photos and record your weight, measurements, and body fat percentage. Check inside including heart rate, blood pressure, cholesterol, coronary risk ratio, your hormone levels, and thyroid. In essence, your post-Transformation progress and results as discussed in Chapter 7.

Consider doing one of the "actual age" assessments that can tell you how old you *really* are. And if you're past forty, I'd even suggest testing your brain age with any of a number of cognitive tests that are becoming increasingly common.

Finally, create a notebook in which you keep your annual Peak Performance Day "scorecards." In a few years you'll have a priceless collection of inspiration to keep going strong for life.

CHAPTER 14

Mastering Motivation

We all want it. Many of us think we need more of it. But just what is motivation? A mix of discipline and desire? A spark that we draw upon whenever needed? While you certainly know what it's like to be motivated as you were during your Transformation, you may not be entirely sure just exactly what motivation is or how to create it. Perhaps you're asking yourself, and wisely so, "How am I going to stay motivated now? How am I going to keep moving forward into greater strength, vitality, and freedom?"

What gets you to do something, let alone to stick with it?

It takes substantial discipline and force to begin a Transformation, and even more fortitude to complete one. Now that your Transformation is behind you, there may be a sense that you can ease up a bit. And while there's certainly some truth to this as far as your body is concerned, this is not the time to let go of the reins. This is a time of great risk, where most people falter after completing a Transformation. You're at a crossroads: Will you choose a life of strength or will you allow it to fade away?

A new challenge awaits you—the challenge of going the distance, sustaining your drive and motivation, and continuing on the path to a life at full strength. Learning how you can take control of the energy that moves you—the force that propels you into action—is the key to effortless sustainability. I'm not talking about the "rah-rah" stuff, but rather the tools and a map, both necessary for you to skillfully navigate the road ahead. Instead of fighting to stay disciplined or relying upon fire and brimstone speeches, in this chapter you will discover how to master motivation, moving beyond discipline to find the joy of being fit and strong, staying engaged for the year ahead and beyond.

Motivation comes from the Latin word *motivus,* meaning "to move." Motivation is the catalyst to action. It's energy for motion—it propels you to *do something.* Without motivation, you have no forward motion in life; your life stagnates. And when you're not growing, you're declining.

More so than any other factor, more than knowledge—even more than the perfect plan—your ability to create, sustain, and renew motivation determines your success in fitness and in life. The perfect plan for certain success is of no use in the absence of the drive to take action. It's through motivation that the rubber hits the road and things get done.

While there are certainly times when it feels great just to have any motivation toward fitness, all motivation is *not* created equal. Some motivation is very intense, others quite subtle. Some motivation has a long shelf life by design, while others pass very quickly. The two basic sources of motivation are *external* and *internal.*

External motivators, the most well known, are commonly referred to as the "carrot and stick." This is the terrain of things we move away from (the stick), like fear, pain, and punishment; and the things we move toward with desire, like the carrot compels the donkey to pull a cart up a mountain. As the name implies, these motivators reside outside of you. They impact your inner experience but stem from beyond your own body and mind. The hallmark of external motivation is that the reward is almost always in the future. External motivators can be strong and highly effective, yet they generally are not sustainable, are easily derailed, and require much effort and discipline.

Internal motivators, on the other hand, arise from within; they're self-generated. Often more powerful, always more sustainable, meaningful, and persistent, internal motivators triumph even in the face of great obstacles. The hallmark of internal motivation is that the reward is found within the activity itself. It's worthy to note that for the large majority of people, the external motivators—the carrot and stick—are the only source of motivation. Hence the reason why the internal motivators are referred to as the "higher reaches" of motivation.

FROM DISCIPLINE TO MASTERY

Contrary to popular myth, a lifetime of fitness is not the product of rock-solid discipline. When you first take on a new challenge in any area of life, it takes a strong compelling reason and considerable discipline simply to engage. Discipline takes great effort and is a short-term strategy—it helps to get you going—but only motivation can keep you going strong. When it comes to sustaining a lifetime of strength and fitness, it's a steady stream of ever-evolving motivation that will carry you to new heights.

When I was thirteen, I decided to learn to play the guitar. I thought it would be a "cool" thing to do. I had this fantasy of playing music. Then I got a dose of reality—while I had ample desire and energy to get started, I came face-to-face with the difficult work: practice. In the absence of progress, I relied on a great amount of discipline to sustain me those first six months. As time went on my efforts began to pay off. Finally I had a noticeable improvement, and just like that, discipline gets a break. In comes in a surge of motivation, fueling a desire to play more. The key was the feedback—the recognition from myself and others that there was improvement began to stoke my desire.

If you've ever had the feeling that getting in shape takes an extraordinary amount of discipline, you're absolutely right—it does, for a short period of time. Furthermore, if you've said, "There's no way I can sustain this type of discipline to stay in shape for life," you're right once again. Thankfully, you don't need to. Discipline carries you only so far because it's short-lived. Motivation carries you the distance. But I'm not just talking about any kind of motivation, I'm talking about the type of motivation that delivers you freedom and sustainability.

Motivation fills the gap between *wanting* and *having* by generating the energy for *doing*. In the absence of motivation, nearly anything you do becomes a great effort—a grueling exercise in discipline. The stages of motivation that follow show you how to move beyond discipline to the higher reaches of motivation, which are not fueled by requirements, but by your passion. When you're doing what you love because you love doing it, everything changes.

Stage 1: Obligation-Based Motivation: "I Should"

People who struggle maintaining a fitness lifestyle tend to lug around a bucket overflowing with obligations in the form of "should." You hear them say they *should* exercise, *should* eat right, and *shouldn't* miss a training session. They should because their doctor told them to; they should because they would have more energy and be in better shape.

This type of external motivation is based on *obligation*. Sustaining it requires discipline—not just your run-of-the-mill discipline, but heaping truckloads of it. Obligation-based motivation is frustrating, draining, and difficult; it's like pushing an enormous stone up a mountain just to have it roll back down again. With each effort, you tell yourself that you "should" get the stone up the mountain. The cycle persists until you're exhausted from the futility of sustaining the task. It's only a matter of time before gravity wins.

Obligation-based motivation is a common point of entry into fitness. It may be enough to get you into the gym or to hire a trainer, but it lacks sustainability. It's the motivational style employed by most dieters, hence the reason 95 percent of them fail.

You'll recognize obligation-based motivation in the framework of the 12 days of Base Camp and the 12 weeks of the TTC. In their pure stand-alone forms, the directions and "to-do's" are a big "should" for you.

Stage 2: Desire-Based Motivation: "I Want To"

Many people train not because it's fun but because they *desire* the body, self-image, confidence, strength, or fitness that their training promises. While still an external source of motivation, at this stage you're moving toward something, not away from it. A positive attraction to a future vision and goals gives desire-based motivation more power and sustainability than obligation-based motivation.

Desire, the next stage in the evolution of motivation, is the way out of the endless cycle of obligation. It operates on the principle that you have to do something to get what you want. You'll stay with your commitments longer and enjoy higher motivation if you use strong and clearly defined goals, as you did in your Transformation.

Moving with focus and intention is a step in the right direction; however, desire-based motivation has an endpoint: the "win" or goals achieved. As such, goals are not the answer to sustainable motivation, but rather, tools to be leveraged along the way. This stage is limited in that the big payoff is almost always in the future, leaving you constantly in pursuit. Many who satisfy their goals and complete a 12-week Transformation quickly revert back. Their loss of motivation a mystery, they recall their experience of transforming fondly and speak of the desire to "get back at it."

You evoke the desire-based motivation in your one-year Vision and TTC goals.

Stage 3: Enjoyment-Based Motivation: "I Love To"

I'd like to invite you back in time to when I first learned to ride a bike. I was an adventurous boy eager to ride and anxious about balancing on two wheels. Yet, I never questioned if I would go for it. I knew my friends would be riding soon if they were not already, and I didn't want to disappoint my parents. Any fear of falling paled in comparison to the obligation I felt to perform.

Enjoyment-Based Motivation

Wanting a sculpted, lean body does not signify enjoyment-based motivation. Having a deep interest and passion to do the activities that naturally lead to such a body is. Enjoying the outcome isn't necessarily enjoying the process of getting there—therein lies a crucial distinction.

It didn't take long for me to get the hang of it, soon cruising around at full speed. I felt as if I were flying! There was no discipline involved—I rode all day long, stopping only when my parents called me home. I didn't ride my bike to get to places, I invented places to go just to *enjoy* the ride.

What do you so love doing that you become lost in the activity itself? It could be anything—reading, cooking, painting, fly-fishing, music, an intimate conversation—it's different for everyone. When you deeply enjoy something, your mind is graced with the presence of the moment.

Stage 3 motivation shatters the "discipline myth," as you're naturally drawn to your fullest expression of life and your true potential. There is no sense of obligation and no need for external pressure.

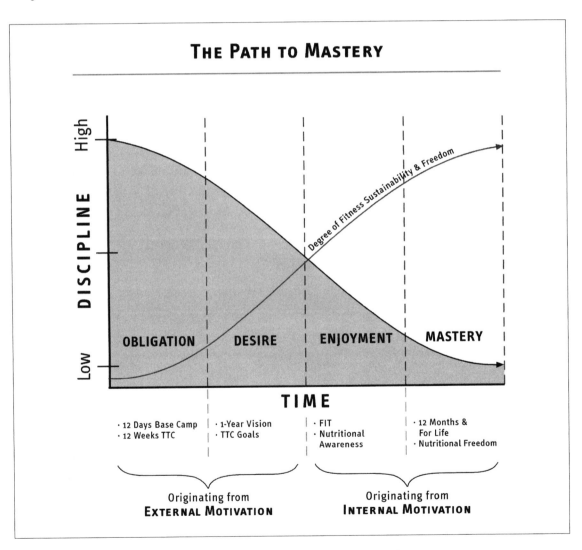

THE PATH TO MASTERY

As enjoyment is found in the depth and focus of your attention, FIT is the perfect practice for fully integrating and engaging your mind and body, producing a deeply enjoyable flow-state experience. With FIT, instead of watching the clock, you'll look back and wonder where the time went.

Stage 4: Mastery: "I'm Inspired, Just Try to Stop Me!"

When an activity ceases to be something you do and becomes a way of life, you begin to experience the pinnacle of freedom: *Mastery.* It arrives unannounced when your practices become integral to your life. At this stage of motivation you do not rely on the first three stages—that's not to say you don't use these types of motivation as stepping-stones; however, you are free from dependence upon them.

Mastery of training frees you from struggling to "get your workout in." You train because that's how you approach life. Your body is strong and vital not because you train; rather, you train to celebrate your strength and vitality. Training is a natural movement for you, just as breathing is a natural spontaneous activity.

In Mastery, you move and take action effortlessly from the perpetual flame of *inspiration.* Here motivation is self-sustaining because it is strengthened by the very actions it motivates. Mastery does not arrive on schedule—it doesn't come in 12 days or 12 weeks. Even the most amazing "after" photo does not assure this freedom and sustainability. Mastery comes only through your steady and full engagement for the 12 months ahead and a consistent annual commitment to strength. It's your path to true freedom and sustainability. Be patient, Mastery takes time.

> Almost without exception, those we know as masters are dedicated to the fundamentals of their calling. They are zealots of practice, connoisseurs of the small, incremental step. At the same time—and here's the paradox—these people are precisely the ones who are likely to challenge previous limits, to take risks for the sake of higher performance, and seem to become obsessive at times in that pursuit. Clearly, for them the key is not either/or, it's both/and.
>
> George Leonard, in his book *Mastery*

MOVING FROM OBLIGATION TO INSPIRATION

1. Trade in Your Obligation for Desire

If you feel as though you *should* take up a training program but it doesn't connect to something you truly desire, don't do it. It's that simple. Just make sure you fully accept and acknowledge the consequences of your actions. If you encounter an obligation that connects with something you truly desire, use it to work for you, but don't rely *exclusively* on obligation-based motivation.

If you're feeling strong energy from this level of motivation, transition through it as fast as possible before your discipline runs out. Get on the short track to changing your obligation into a desire. Get focused on the future, on a result you truly want.

Tip: Leverage a trainer or training partner to provide a positive obligation, but be sure to stay focused on what you truly desire.

Examples:

BEFORE: **OBLIGATION**	AFTER: **DESIRE**
"*I should* be healthy"	"*I want* to be strong"
"*I should* get in better shape"	"*I want* to look ten years younger"

2. Find Clarity and Inspire Desire

Motivation is as strong as it is clear. In the absence of clarity and focus, motivation's energy turns to frustration. Take the time to figure out exactly what you truly desire (your carrot). Look within: What is a vision, goal, or destination worthy of your time, attention, and energy? Once you are clear about what you truly desire, take steps to educate yourself about what it will take to attain it. Use the skills discussed in Chapter 6 to fuel your motivation.

Tip: Engage in friendly competition. Few things activate our innate desire like competitive fire. A friendly Transformation challenge can elicit powerful motivation to help you achieve things you would not otherwise contemplate. Even in competition your aim should not be to surpass others but to constantly surpass your own previous best. Competition can inspire your greater potential.

Tip: Measure your progress; use this feedback to fuel desire.

3. Learn to Love the Process

The most important step in mastering motivation, yet in many ways the most difficult, is learning to love the process. If you're committed to growing beyond the carrot and stick to a truly sustainable form of motivation, then you must learn to fall in love with training itself and not just the results. Patience, commitment, and persistence are all essential ingredients; however, ultimately you must aim for joy, and you'll discover—in the least expected of moments—Mastery.

Connect with your passion—what truly *moves* and *inspires* you. As you discover how to love the training leading you to the goals that matter most, you will transform discipline into freedom, struggle into grace, and willpower into passion.

Tip: Avoid the struggle between where you are now and where you "should be." Embrace where you are now. This is your gateway to Mastery.

Tip: Be patient. Be consistent.

Strength for the Journey

Your life is a journey, and motivation is the fuel that keeps you going strong.

Sustaining motivation is vital to your continued growth along the path of life, and it can be tricky to navigate. Over the course of weeks, months, and years, motivation rises and falls. It will come on strong and wane in seasons to follow. At times you may find yourself struggling with discipline and obligation, other times you'll be soaring with inspiration.

Freedom is found in the higher reaches of motivation, but the true power is in the mix—an ever-changing blend of the stages of motivation. The path to your ever-evolving personal best lies in your acceptance of what is and your commitment to confidently move forward. It's the delicate balance of tension between these two points—where you are now and where you're going—from which motivation propels you into action.

CHAPTER 15

Share the Strength

Why is it that some people change their bodies and others Transform their lives? What is it that ignites life's brilliance deep within?

By all accounts there are many different stories of Transformation success, and those who continue to evolve and Transform year after year hold a secret—a universal truth shared by all who have made this momentous leap. I want to leave you with an inside look at this secret that not only sustains your physical strength but will have you living a life of meaning and impact.

The secret of reaching your potential is in the unlimited capacity of body, mind, heart, and soul that can only be found deep within, where your true strength arises. Most people never know the true depth of their strength because they've never been tested or pushed to find out what they're made of—physically, mentally, spiritually.

When you discover this unshakable belief in your strength, you begin to open to what you're here for *and* can do with this lifetime. Ultimately, the measure of your life is in the difference you make in this world—in your impact on others. Doing more, being more, and giving more calls upon your reservoir of strength. Only with considerable capacity can you be in a position to do the most for others and be of the greatest service to those who mean the most in your life.

You began your Transformation with a commitment to strength as a guiding value. You were tested and no doubt at times felt anything but strong. As you came to recognize your strength, you brought your potential to the surface and now stand forever changed, to a new way of being.

The last few months have been vital to awakening your strength. You could liken it to the journey made by the characters in *The Wizard of Oz*. They all believed the Wizard held the power to fulfill their deepest wishes, to give them what they believed missing. After following "The Yellow Brick Road," the Scarecrow, the Lion, the Tin Man, and Dorothy discovered that what they each sought, they already possessed. For them to have lived without making the journey not only would have meant the tragic loss of a classic movie, but to live without the realization of their true gifts.

Like the characters in *The Wizard of Oz*, you've come to discover the strength you already possessed. Your journey has helped you cultivate that strength: revealing your greater capacity, forging your body and mind strong.

Now it's your turn to be the Wizard, to reach from within, to share the strength you've uncovered with others and to help them embark on their own journeys. As the practice of training and eating right strengthens and enlivens your body, so does the act of contribution—big or small—nourish your soul.

Share your energy, time, and passion freely. Contribute your knowledge, not just of this program, but of all your accumulated wisdom. In your service and contribution to others is where both you and those around you receive the greatest returns. When you share your strength, you get stronger; everyone gets stronger.

How strong are you? How will you lift the world? How will you be a beacon of strength for others? These questions are of utmost importance. As my father's passing taught me, it is wise not to assume we possess more time than what we have here. Our opportunity to make our mark resides in this moment, and the clock is ticking. Every one of us has a time limit to fulfill our destiny. Don't be one who waits for the final buzzer to start to really live. Yesterday is a memory and tomorrow is a dream. Today is the day to make your mark—to make a difference.

BURN BRIGHT

There's something deeply entrancing about the magical power of a flame; the point of ignition is the purest, rawest form of Transformation. It's to witness the moment when something truly transforms and releases its energy in a glorious dance, becoming something else. We're attracted to this power, we fear it, but our fascination with fire never disappears because of the life we see in it. Don't believe me? Go take a look. You'll find yourself in rapture as the flames of your fire begin to dance.

A fire resides within each of us. This fire is your life, the source of energy that fuels your freedom, strength, and vitality. You are a living, breathing Transformation moment to moment.

Some people would rather not see it—to do so is to know what they are capable of; to see the strength, the power, the force that is inside, is to have responsibility. Instead they turn away. Their flame is ignored. Yet others stoke their flame. They radiate that which has no limits, they are the most contagious and burn the brightest. You can see it; it's as if they are light themselves. *Brilliance* is the word we use to describe these people as they burn with the brightness of the sun. In recognition, we take them in with the same fascination with which we look at fire in all of its grace and elegance.

The fire inside lives within the many hundreds of thousands of Transformations I've seen. You ignited the flame in your Transformation—now it's time to fan the flame. You are made to ignite and burn with a higher luminosity than you already have; the brighter your fire burns, the more fuel it attracts and the more people you will inspire—and the greater your impact.

> *To burn brightly is to live fully.*
> *To be alive is to make a difference.*
> *To act in service is to love.*
> *To love is to have strength.*
> *To share your strength is to burn bright.*

Find the spark and ignite your flame. Burn brightly for yourself, your family, your community, your country, your world. Don't delay, we're all counting on you. Live every day to the fullest and create your legacy. Making your impact in the world is your destination. Step into every moment with all your courage and strength.

This is your life. Shine like the sun.

Welcome to the *beginning* of the *best* of your life.

Epilogue

As your journey to a life of strength continues, you will experience a breakthrough: when your deepest desires—what you truly want—align with what is best for you, your family, the world. To discover this strength and clarity is the beginning to a life of freedom. Only this is not the freedom we may have dreamed of in our youth—the freedom to avoid the realities of life—but rather freedom found in the strength and courage to be fully with life, as it is. It's not swimming in the ocean of life but surfing its waves—always steadily, skillfully moving forward with ease— being all that you are in each moment.

Now I challenge you to share your strength—and to share your stories of strength with me. I look forward to hearing how you've Transformed your body, your life, and the lives of others. Please share your stories. You can e-mail me at shawn@ShareTheStrength.com.

I've been honored to serve as your guide to a lifetime of strength.

Yours, in Strength,

Shawn Phillips

Questions and Answers

Q: Who really gets the most out of the *Strength for Life* program?

A: The *Strength for Life* program is not age- or gender-specific. It's just as important for an 18-year-old to eat well and train as it is for an 88-year-old.

Additionally, stamina and flexibility are essential elements for energizing the body and mind. And when it comes to strengthening your body with sound, proven training, Focus Intensity Training provides the extra boost allowing the training to be short, sweet, maximally effective, and most important, *enjoyable*—so it's nearly perfect for a man or woman of any age.

Use good judgment when starting your *Strength for Life* program. Regardless of your age, if you've not been regularly exercising or, as I like to say, *training,* you will want to engage the program in a gradual manner.

Q: I'm on the road for nearly two weeks each month; how can I bring my strength training with me?

A: Traveling presents a challenge because it disrupts your normal routines. And, for many, travel of any sort is a reason to toss aside all commitments, especially when it comes to eating and training. As a highly seasoned traveler, you no doubt no longer think of travel as a treat. It's part of your work, your responsibility. And as such, you're likely to enjoy the freedom you'll find in bringing your Transformation on the road. It brings a new challenge and texture to your travel.

Thankfully, many hotels have adequate gyms or relationships with nearby facilities. Be sure to ask when making reservations. Or, if you have a membership in a national fitness chain, try to arrange your hotel accommodations nearby. Use what you can find in the hotel, enjoy the gym, or find the fire escape and run the stairs. This is a reliable way to get a workout in when the weather prohibits you from going out. Be creative, resourceful, and committed.

Q: How do I eat healthy on the road?

A: The key is planning and staying committed to your Transformation progress. On almost any restaurant menu, you can find a lean protein source and vegetables. Don't be afraid to ask to substitute healthy carbohydrate choices (e.g., veggies, brown or wild rice) for french fries. My secret weapon when I travel is my Full Strength blender bottle: In just seconds, I can mix a Full Strength Premium Nutrition Shake. This is a perfect solution given the fast-paced tempo of business travel, and it beats raiding the hotel minibar or gift shop candy aisle.

While going mobile is not ideal for a Transformation, if it's what you've got, go full out with it and you will succeed. When on the road, more than ever it's up to you. Bring your focus and discipline into play and you can succeed anywhere, and when you do it on the road, the confidence boost alone will be worth the commitment.

Q: How do I measure my body fat percentage?

A: I suggest using a simple pair of calipers and selecting one or two trouble areas on your body to measure weekly throughout your Transformation. Make sure your measurements are taken on the same spot on your body each time. You're losing fat if the number is going down, gaining fat if the number is going up. Your calipers will come with a specific set of instructions to guide you. Alternatively, you can have your trainer perform and track these measurements for you.

What matters most is not your body fat percentage but your relative change in body fat as the weeks go by. It's not where you're at, it's where you're headed.

Q: How do I know when I'm gaining muscle and losing fat?

A: The first clue you're gaining muscle and losing fat is you're gaining weight but getting smaller. Your caliper tests will reveal a smaller number. If you use a tape to measure your waist, hips, or trouble areas regularly, you'll also have this affirmation of your progress. You will also feel it and see it in certain clothes. Once tight-fitting jeans begin to feel roomier, shirts and blouses begin to fit differently. These are all cues that you're losing fat.

As you begin to shape and sculpt your body lean, you'll gain strength. You may not necessarily feel stronger on all your exercises, but during your TTC your strength will increase. Over time your muscle tone and definition will reveal themselves in the mirror. This is your cue that you're gaining muscle.

Q: How do I use FIT in my stretching and in my cardio?

A: While FIT is the practice of intertwining peaks of intense focus with periods of deep and full recovery as you deepen your practice, you will come to see that the entire practice resides on a stream of presence and awareness. So, while your cardio and stretching sessions require a different type of concentration and intensity, you will begin to bring forward this stream of presence into the rest of your training. In cardio you may find yourself focused on your breath or finding a rhythm and pace that keeps you in the room, not out of it. For stretching, try breathing into the muscle being stretched, focusing on the movement of energy inside that muscle. You will find many of the mind–body integration benefits of FIT in most yoga practices. Be as present to your cardio and stretching as you are to your biceps under full contraction.

Q: Can I listen to music when I'm doing FIT?

A: While you can listen to anything you wish while doing FIT, including the sound of a jackhammer crushing concrete if that's your thing, I urge you to give yourself at least a solid four to five weeks of peace and quiet in your training before you crank up your favorite tunes. Consider that you are training your mind—completely rewiring its ability to focus and staying present in the spaces between—which is best done in quiet, where you can deal only with the considerable noise your mind is going to make.

After about four weeks, you are free to bring music back into your training, as many find that music helps them stay focused and present, preventing distracting conversations in the gym. The best music choices are those with consistent, steady beats and not a lot of vocals. But if it's a song with lyrics you've heard many times, that's okay too. The bottom line is that you want music that's going to seem like background noise, not something that will consume your focus.

Q: What if I miss a workout?

A: If you miss a workout one day, the best thing to do is to "stack" your training the next day. If you miss a Tuesday workout, stick to your strength training session on Wednesday, and add your HIIT and abs (it's only an additional 30 minutes). If you miss a strength day, push it to the next cardio day but start with strength and then finish with cardio even if this is a cardio lead day (Tuesday and Friday). But the best solution is to not miss a day—not during the 12 short weeks of the TTC. If it happens, it happens, but if it happens twice, you're wise to reflect on your reasons—and go back to see if your goals are drawing you forward.

Q: Can I strength-train and do my cardio on the same day? If so, what should I do first?

A: The TTC schedule is designed to optimize your gains by focusing on either strength or cardio each day. Whenever you double dip by doing both on the same day, you're going to lose *some* impact. Yet, should you choose to stack these two in your "off-peak seasons," as many will, you should always do your strength training first.

This is because strength calls on the availability of a fast-acting fuel called glycogen. If you do your cardio first, you'll burn up much of the available glycogen, leaving your muscles weaker and less able to reach Peak Intensity in your strength training. Another upside to this order is that strength training utilizes much of the glycogen most readily available, thus requiring the following cardio session to draw upon other fuel for creating more energy—and much of this energy may come from fat stores.

Q: Do I need a training partner? Do I need a spotter working with dumbbells?

A: Having a training partner can bring many advantages. However, it's not at all critical that you have a spotter or train with anyone. Dumbbells can minimize your risk of injury once you've learned the proper form and technique, as you can push yourself to your edge and safely lower the weights to your sides without worrying to rerack a barbell. I recommend a spotter as you're learning, but as you master strength training with dumbbells, a spotter becomes less important.

The right training partner can keep you committed to your program and offer support. But it's by no means necessary. Some people make the mistake of chatting too much with their training partner, extending the training sessions and making them less effective.

Q: Does the *Strength for Life* program improve my balance?

A: Any sort of regular physical movement and exercise will help strengthen your body and the connection between your body and mind—what's called your "kinesthetic" or body awareness. Strength training will get you more in touch with your body, rewire your brain, and improve your ability to move and balance yourself. This may not translate immediately to international success on the balance beam, but rest assured that you'll have a much more solid ground in everything you do every day.

Q: What if I get hungry between meals?

A: When you start eating five balanced meals each day, it's likely that you'll feel that you're eating too much food at first. After a few weeks of training, your metabolism will speed up and you'll find yourself with more of a healthy appetite, but this usually comes like clockwork within the three-hour time frame when your next meal is due.

Still, there will be times when you're hungry before your next meal. I offer you three suggestions. First, drink some water, perhaps you're thirsty. Second, if the water doesn't satiate the hunger and you're close to a meal, eat. Then shift your other meal plans accordingly. Finally, if your meal is an hour or more away, add a meal and take note of your last meal and how much you ate; perhaps you're underfeeding yourself. Remember, five meals may *sound* like a lot at first, but your *Strength for Life* training keeps your metabolism red hot, and you may find yourself needing more nutrients.

Q: Can I use resistance bands instead of weights?

A: Weights are one of the best ways to provide resistance to help you gain strength, build lean muscle, and reshape your body; however, there are other forms of resistance that you can use given the appropriate situation.

Bands are a good way to introduce resistance to your workouts if you're in a bind on the road and unable to make it to a gym, as they're highly portable. Using body weight exercises in conjunction with resistance bands while leveraging the powerful focus of your mind with FIT enables you to get a great workout outside of the gym or your home. While good resistance bands have many benefits and even more uses, I'm not suggesting you trade in your dumbbells for resistance bands. Gravity is a much more reliable force than rubber tubing.

Q: Can I use an energy bar for one of my meals each day?

A: I find the use of the term "energy" in association with many nutrition bars and even many sports drinks to be one of the greatest misnomers in advertising and culture today. Energy is created in the body through the use of balanced, nourishing meals.

The food we eat can and should be a source of energy, but the sort of fuel that most energy bars and sports drinks are filled with are most likely robbing you of the energy you most want—unless your body is being worked extensively and is in desperate need for sugars and other fast-acting carbohydrates.

Bars are best for convenience when you're on an outing where you need the extra burst of carbohydrates and something easy to keep in your pocket. The *best* of the bars are designed with natural sources and are well built for a strenuous hike or long bike ride, but not the sort of nutrition you need in your car or at your desk. They're also good for what I call a "better bad choice" when your options are missing a meal or eating a triple burger with cheese, but don't make them a reliable source of daily nutrition.

Bars are simply not a sound source of daily nutrition, nor should they be considered a meal.

Instead, eat foods that nourish your body and mind and provide hours of energy and strength. Use your strategies from Chapter 10. You can do better than energy bars with a little planning ahead of time. Your body and mind will reflect the quality of your choice.

Q: How can I best follow the *Strength for Life* nutrition plan while adhering to a vegan diet?

A: As both the vegan and vegetarian lifestyles are becoming increasingly popular, I fully expect, and encourage, anyone endeavoring to adopt either to educate themselves with some of the many quality publications and guides, because there are some important things you should know.

As most vegans and vegetarians are well aware, it's important that you enjoy an abundance and variety of vegetables, grains, and salads to ensure adequate intake of vitamins and minerals. It's common for both vegans and vegetarians to have deficiencies in vitamin B_{12}, iron, zinc (especially for men), calcium, and even creatine. Most are found in abundance (and some exclusively) in meats. Many vegans find themselves craving sugar when protein is deficient.

As for the ever vital source of proteins, a few of the best include: raw nuts, seeds, soy, tofu, miso, almond milk, soy milk, tempeh, beans, lentils, and nut butters. There are also an increasing number of proteins available that originate from whole grains, including buckwheat, hemp, chickpeas, and rice. In the cross-over vegetable-proteins, you'll find quinoa, millet, amaranth, and whole-grain brown rice. It's important to diversify your protein sources.

In terms of the structure, meal frequency, and balance, all of these apply whatever your choice of diet.

Food List

PROTEINS	VEGETABLES	FRUITS
beef and buffalo (lean, organic)*	alfalfa sprouts	apple
chicken (organic, skinless)	artichoke	applesauce—unsweetened
dried beans	arugula	apricot
egg whites	asparagus	avocado
egg yolks* (organic)	beets	banana
fresh fish:	bell peppers	blackberries
cod	black beans	blueberries
flounder	bok choy	cherries
tilapia	broccoli	grapefruit
halibut	brussels sprouts	kiwi
mackerel	cabbage	mango
salmon	carrots	melon
tuna	cauliflower	nectarine
garbanzo beans	celery	orange
lamb	cucumber	papaya
lentils	endive	peach
low-fat cottage cheese	green or yellow beans	pear
low-fat yogurt*	greens—mustard	pineapple
non-fat yogurt	jicama	plum
tofu	kale	prune
turkey (skinless)	leeks	raspberries
	lettuce	strawberries (organic)
	mushrooms	watermelon
	onions	
	radishes	
	rutabaga	
	sea vegetables (seaweed, kelp, nori)	
	snow peas	
	spinach	
	squash—summer and winter	
	sweet or baked potatoes	
	tomatoes	
	turnips	
	water chestnuts	
	yams	
	zucchini	

*In moderation

GRAINS	NUTS, SEEDS, OILS	BEVERAGES	NUTRITION SHAKE

amaranth
cream of rice
millet
oatmeal
puffed rice
Quinoa
Quinoa pasta*
rice (brown, wild)
rice bread
rice cakes, rice
   crackers
rice milk
rice pasta
spelt bread or wrap
whole-grain pasta*
whole wheat bread*
	almond butter*
	almonds
	cashews
	flax oil
	ground flaxseeds
	hazelnuts
	natural peanut butter*
	olive oil—cold-pressed,
	   extra virgin
	pecans
	safflower oil
	sunflower oil
	walnut oil
	walnuts
		cranberry juice*
		   (unsweetened, or-
		   ganic)
		pomegranate juice*
		water
		green tea
		herbal tea
		skim milk (organic)
		soy milk
			Full Strength

*In moderation			

Nutrition Tracker

STRENGTH FOR LIFE DAILY NUTRITION & AWARENESS PRACTICE

NAME _____

DATE _____   WEEK _____

	FOODS and BEVERAGES CONSUMED	BODY + MIND STATE	WATER/TIME
MEAL #1 Time: AM [ ] PM [ ]			
MEAL #2 Time: AM [ ] PM [ ]			
MEAL #3 Time: AM [ ] PM [ ]			
MEAL #4 Time: AM [ ] PM [ ]			
MEAL #5 Time: AM [ ] PM [ ]			
OTHER Time: AM [ ] PM [ ]			

STRENGTH FOR LIFE DAILY NUTRITION & AWARENESS PRACTICE

NAME _____

DATE _____ WEEK _____

	FOODS and BEVERAGES CONSUMED	BODY + MIND STATE	WATER/TIME
MEAL #1 Time: AM [ ] PM [ ]			
MEAL #2 Time: AM [ ] PM [ ]			
MEAL #3 Time: AM [ ] PM [ ]			
MEAL #4 Time: AM [ ] PM [ ]			
MEAL #5 Time: AM [ ] PM [ ]			
OTHER Time: AM [ ] PM [ ]			

Exercise Guide

Here's a list of the basic strength training exercises you will perform throughout your 12-week Transformation—all very sound, rewarding, and straightforward. Nevertheless, I've provided easy-to-follow instructions to guide you through each movement.

Proper form is necessary to deliver optimal results and protect you from injury. As such, I encourage you to study the photos for your start/finish positions and midpoint, as well as pick up some helpful tips on how to get the most out of each exercise.

Remember, though, it's not the *what* but the *how* that creates the enjoyment, produces the greatest satisfaction, and allows you to get the most from your training in the least amount of time. For that reason I also offer you some suggestions on where to place your focus and concentration throughout each exercise.

Be sure to deepen your concentration with each rep, in every set you perform; recall the Focus Intensity Index from Chapter 11 as a reference.

The primary muscle group being trained in this exercise is your chest, with your shoulders and triceps in a supportive engagement.

Starting Position: With feet flat on the floor, lie back on a bench while holding dumbbells in each hand at the outside edges of your shoulders. Be sure to keep the weights chest high. Your palms face toward your feet as your elbows bend at a 90-degree angle. Keep your head on the bench and your lower back flat–don't arch.

The Exercise: Press the weight up while you breathe out, keeping the weight directly over your chest. Lower the weight in a horizontal plane with your shoulders as you inhale, keeping your elbows and weights in line with your chest. Do not lock your elbows at the top of the movement, then lower the weights slowly. Momentarily pause at the bottom before pressing the weights back up.

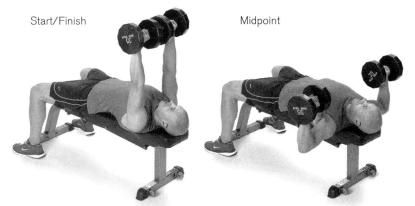

Start/Finish   Midpoint

Tips: Control the weight all the way up, slightly touching the weights together. Do not clank the weights forcefully together at the top of this movement.

Focal Point: Create the strongest contraction in your chest and triceps. As the intensity builds, keep your breathing steady and in rhythm with each repetition. Guide your attention to your focal point throughout the set.

Don't Do: Don't allow your elbows and the weights to float past your shoulders toward your head. Keep your shoulders and the weights in line.

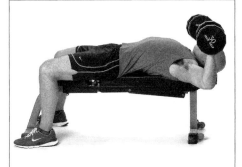

The primary muscle group being trained in this exercise is your chest, with your shoulders in a supportive engagement.

Starting Position: Sit on the edge of a bench with a dumbbell in each hand. Lie back keeping the dumbbells close to your chest. Keep your palms facing each other, your hips and lower back firmly grounded on the bench, and your feet flat on the floor.

The Exercise: Begin with elbows slightly bent and lower the dumbbells out to the sides, making a T with your arms and your torso. Don't let your arms go below the bench. Then press the dumbbells up in an arc, as if you're giving someone a hug. Lightly touch the weights together above your chest and slowly return the dumbbells to the starting position. Be sure to exhale on the way up and inhale on the way down.

Tips: Don't allow your hands to lower below your shoulders. This can place additional stress on the shoulder joint. Drive the weights together from your chest and avoid using your arms to move the weights together.

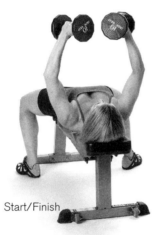

Start/Finish

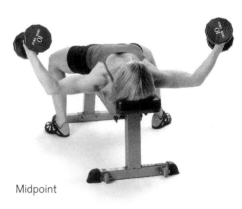

Midpoint

Focal Point: Draw your attention directly into your chest throughout this exercise, keeping your breathing steady and consistent.

Don't Do: Keep the weights in line with your elbows and shoulders and don't allow your arms to rotate.

The primary muscle group used in this exercise is your shoulders.

Starting Position: Stand upright, with your feet about shoulder width apart. Start with the dumbbells at your sides.

The Exercise: While exhaling, raise the arms to a point where they're even with the shoulders, palms facing down to the floor. Keep your arms almost perfectly straight, forming a T with your torso. Keep your knees slightly bent while performing the entire range of motion. Pause for a moment at the top and lower the weights slowly while inhaling.

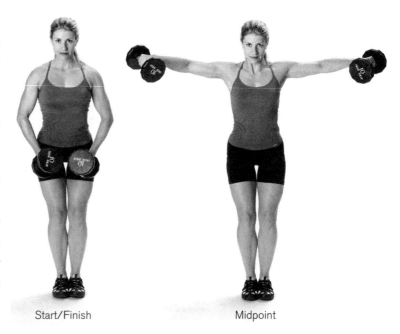

Start/Finish   Midpoint

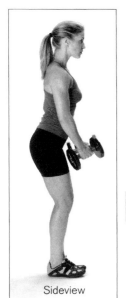

Sideview

✓ **Tips:** It's important to keep your palms turned downward as you lift the dumbbells, to isolate your shoulder muscles. Make sure you lean slightly forward throughout this movement, lifting the dumbbells slowly rather than *swinging* them.

Focal Point: Steadily press the weights up while rolling the shoulder blades toward one another. Focus on creating the fullest, most complete contraction of your shoulder muscles.

The primary muscles in this exercise are your triceps.

Starting Position: Place one knee and one hand comfortably on a bench, keeping your back straight and shoulders and hips parallel with the ground. Pick up a dumbbell with your free hand, keeping the weight parallel with the bench. Exhale on the way up and inhale on the way down.

The Exercise: Pull the dumbbell up, stopping when your elbow is directly at your side. Without changing the position of your elbow throughout the rest of the exercise, slowly extend your arm until it's straight and your triceps are fully contracted. Briefly pause with your arm straight and slowly lower the weight. Repeat with the other arm.

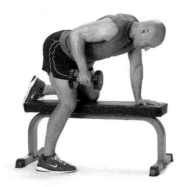 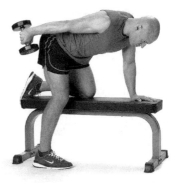

Start/Finish   Midpoint

 Tips: Keeping your elbow directly at your side is critical for this movement. Maintaining proper form is key. Avoid any swinging motion with the dumbbell. Slowly lower the weight until your hand is directly under your elbow before lifting the weight back up again.

Focal Point: Focus on maintaining a contracted muscle, without relaxing, throughout this entire range of motion.

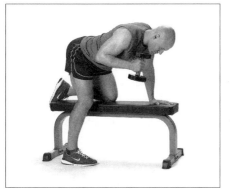

Don't Do: Don't allow your elbow to drop down from your side, and do not swing the weight toward your shoulder before beginning your next rep.

The primary muscles in this exercise are your biceps.

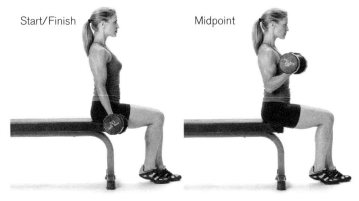

Start/Finish   Midpoint

Starting Position: From a seated position, hold two dumbbells, allowing your arms to naturally rest at your sides, palms facing forward (if standing, stand with feet shoulder width apart).

The Exercise: Lift the weights slowly up toward your chest, keeping your elbows directly at your sides from start to finish. Contract the biceps muscle as hard as you can at the top and hold it for a count of one. Then lower the weights for a count of two. One of the best ways to increase the effectiveness of this exercise is to let the weight down slowly. Exhale on the way up and inhale on the way down.

Focal Point

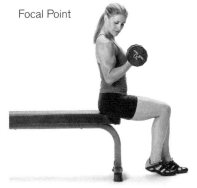

✔ **Tips:** To optimize the intensity in your arms, avoid moving the elbows forward or backward. Keeping your elbows from moving will help you isolate your biceps and increase the effectiveness of your training. Keep your back straight and, if standing, knees slightly bent.

Focal Point: Center your attention directly on your bicep. Generate the fullest, tightest contraction at the top of this movement. Maintain a strong contraction of your bicep as you lower the weight.

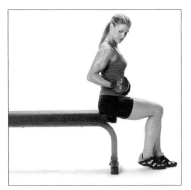

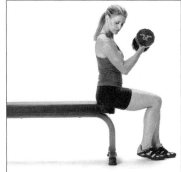

🚫 **Don't Do:** Don't allow your elbow to shift backward or forward during each rep.

The primary muscle groups in this exercise are your quadriceps, hamstrings, and glutes.

Starting Position: Stand with feet together, toes pointed forward, with a dumbbell in each hand. Keep your back straight, shoulders and hips squared, and chin up.

The Exercise: Step forward with the right foot. While inhaling, bend at the knees and lower the hips until the left knee is just a few inches off the floor and your front leg is at a 90-degree angle. Exhaling, push up and back with the right leg and bring your feet together, raising your body to the starting point. Complete all reps with your right leg before continuing to your left leg.

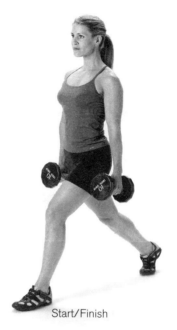
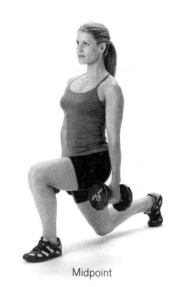

Start/Finish   Midpoint

Tips: Make sure that your front knee never moves beyond your ankle, as this can cause strain on the knee joint. Also make sure that both feet are pointed straight forward. Use the front leg to primarily lift/lower the weight, allowing the back leg to be used for maintaining balance.

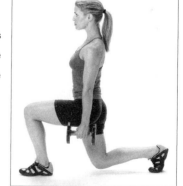

Focal Point: Focus your attention within the deep muscles of your thigh, both front (quads) and back (hamstrings). Feel the intensity in utilizing both regions of these large muscle groups as you fully contract each area during both concentric and eccentric movements.

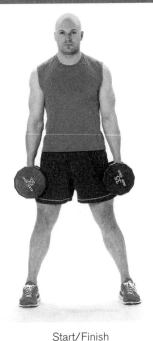

The primary muscle groups used during this exercise are your quadriceps and hamstrings, with your calf muscles in a supportive engagement.

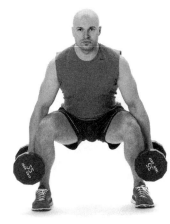

Starting Position: Stand with your feet shoulder width apart. Hold two dumbbells at your sides with palms facing in.

The Exercise: Keep your shoulders back, your back straight, and head upright; bend your legs at the knees and lower your hips until your thighs are parallel with the floor. Then, pushing down into your heels and the balls of your feet, lift yourself back up to the starting position. Breathe into your belly on the way down and forcefully exhale as you stand up.

Start/Finish   Midpoint

Tips: Be sure to keep your chin up and your eyes straight ahead (or looking gently up) to help you maintain proper balance throughout this exercise.

Focal Point: Focus your attention keenly on proper form—specifically, the alignment of your spine—throughout this movement. Feel the strong contraction of the quadriceps muscles as you lower your body down, and of the hamstrings as you press your body back up.

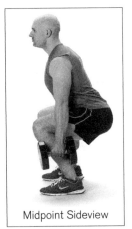

Midpoint Sideview

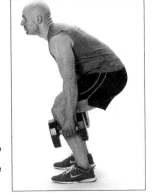

Don't Do: Don't allow your lower back to round forward to lower the weights. Keep your back flat and sit down into the squat to lower the weights.

The primary muscle group used in this exercise is your hamstrings, with your glutes in a supportive engagement.

Starting Position: Stand straight with feet shoulder width apart and a dumbbell in each hand resting in front of your hips/thighs, with your palms facing toward the front of your legs.

The Exercise: Bend forward at the hips and slowly lower the dumbbells in front of you until the weights almost touch the floor (or until your back starts to roll forward). Keep the back straight and legs straight (but not locked at the knees) throughout the exercise. While concentrating on the muscles in the back of your legs, raise your upper body and the weights to the starting position.

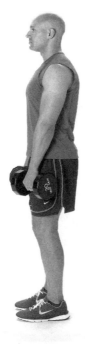

Start/Finish

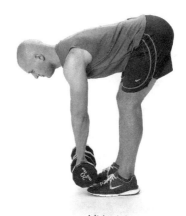

Midpoint

 Tips: Keep your hands close to your shins, arch your back slightly, and stick your chest out throughout the exercise to keep the weight supported by your hamstrings.

Focal Point: Feel your hamstring muscles lengthen and stretch as you lower the weight. Then initiate the upward movement by contracting your hamstring and glute muscles. A secondary point of focus for this exercise is your glutes. Once you return to the standing position, focus on contracting your glutes by rolling your hips under, heightening the contraction before beginning your next repetition.

The primary muscle groups used during this exercise are your quadriceps and hamstrings, with your calf muscles in a supportive engagement.

Starting Position: Hold one dumbbell in front of you, as illustrated. Stand with your feet shoulder width apart. Next, step each foot out to your side approximately 6 to 12 inches. As you place each foot out to your side, move it out at a 45-degree angle.

Start/Finish

Midpoint

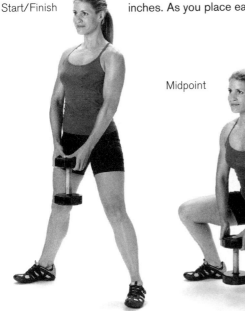

The Exercise: Keep your shoulders back, your back straight, and head upright; bend your legs at the knees and lower your hips until your thighs are parallel with the floor as you allow your knees to stay in line with your feet. Then, pushing down into your heels and the balls of your feet, lift yourself back up to the starting position. Breathe into your belly on the way down and forcefully exhale as you stand up.

Tips: Be sure to keep your chin up and your eyes straight ahead (or looking gently up) to help you maintain proper balance throughout this exercise.

Focal Point: Focus your attention keenly on proper form—specifically, the alignment of your spine—throughout this movement. Feel the strong contraction of the quadriceps muscles as you lower your body down, and of the hamstrings as you press your body back up.

The primary muscle group used in this exercise is your calves.

Starting Position: Stand with the ball of your right foot resting on a step and hold a dumbbell in your right hand, while holding onto something for balance with the left hand. Slightly bend your left leg and allow it to float comfortably next to your right leg without resting it on anything.

The Exercise: While inhaling, lower your right heel as far as possible, stretching your calf muscles at the bottom of the movement. Exhaling, press up onto your toes as far as possible, contracting the calf muscles. Momentarily pause at the top of this movement before lowering yourself down. After you've completed all of the reps for your right leg, switch legs.

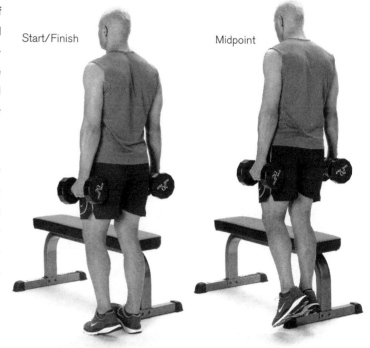

Start/Finish   Midpoint

Tips: Keep your knee slightly bent throughout this movement and avoid any bouncing motion. Also be sure to keep your foot straight, not allowing it to turn either inward or out.

Focal Point: Drive yourself up as far as possible onto the ball of your foot, creating the strongest, fullest contraction. Strive to achieve the absolute highest point and strongest contraction with each and every repetition.

The primary muscle group used in this exercise is your back, with your shoulders and arms in a supportive engagement.

Starting Position: Place one knee and one hand on a flat bench. Your knee on the bench is placed under (or close to) your hip, and your hand on the bench is placed under (or close to) your shoulder. Plant your opposite foot firmly on the ground with a slight bend in your knee. Place a dumbbell on the floor under your free arm.

The Exercise: Start lifting the dumbbell up by squeezing your shoulder blades together, then pulling the weight toward the middle of your rib cage with your arm as you exhale. Keep your shoulders parallel to the floor. Pause slightly at the top of the movement before slowly lowering the weight as you inhale. Keep your elbow close to your body and your back flat throughout this movement.

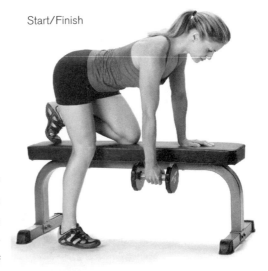

Start/Finish

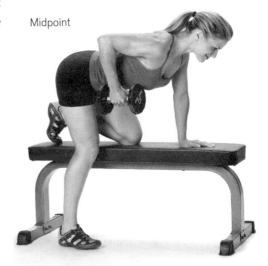

Midpoint

Tips: Do not rotate your torso or head as you lift the dumbbell. To help minimize rotation, thus isolating the muscles in the back of the shoulder more effectively, you can gently turn your head toward your support arm, tucking your chin into your shoulder. Do not hunch or round your back, and do not allow your bicep and arm to be the central focus.

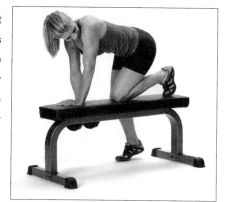

Focal Point: Contract the muscles in your back, tightly squeezing your shoulder blades together. Focus your attention here throughout the exercise.

Don't Do: Don't turn your chest and head upward while rowing the dumbbell up. Keep looking down throughout the entire range of motion and keep your shoulders parallel with the floor.

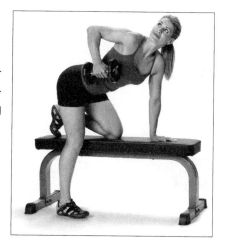

The primary muscle group used in this exercise is your back, with your chest, triceps, and abs in a supportive engagement.

Starting Position: Lie perpendicular across a flat bench with only your upper back on the bench. Your feet are approximately shoulder width apart and flat on the floor. Push your hips up so they are almost parallel with your shoulders. Hold the dumbbell with flattened hands against the inside upper plate of one end straight above your chest.

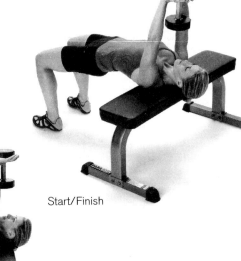

Start/Finish

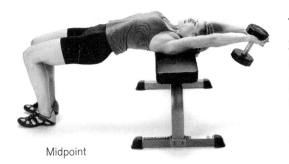

Midpoint

The Exercise: Slowly arch the dumbbell out above your head, keeping your arms almost straight, and breathe in. Stop when the dumbbell is horizontal with your head (or slightly lower if shoulder flexibility allows). Exhale as you slowly raise the dumbbell, bringing the weight above your forehead. Slightly pause, then lower the weight, beginning your next repetition.

Tips: You should feel your hamstrings working to maintain the proper posture of keeping your hips up throughout the entire range of motion.

 Focal Point: Keeping your core tight while contracting your back, chest, and shoulder muscles while at the same time extending the dumbbell out, making a large arc with your arms.

 Don't Do: Do not allow your hips to drop down at any point in this exercise.

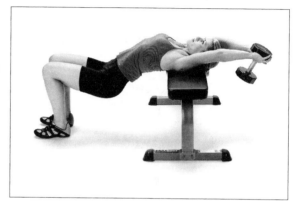

The primary muscles used in this exercise are the back of your shoulders (rear delts), with your upper back muscles in a supportive engagement.

Starting Position: Sit at the edge of a bench with a dumbbell in each hand. Lean your torso over your legs while keeping your back flat. Allow the dumbbells to hang down at your ankles.

Start/Finish

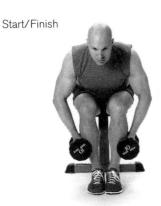

Midpoint

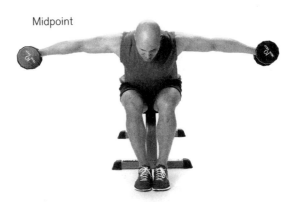

The Exercise: Raise the dumbbells directly out away from your legs, opening up your chest and squeezing your shoulder blades together. Keep your palms facing down throughout this exercise. Keep a slight bend in your arms as you complete each repetition.

✓ **Tips:** Lead with your elbows as you begin each repetition, allowing your wrists and the dumbbells to follow.

Focal Point: Focus on tightly contracting upper back muscles, drawing your shoulder blades together.

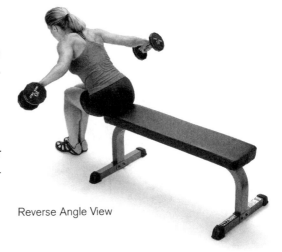

Reverse Angle View

The primary muscles trained in this exercise are your triceps, the back of your upper arm.

Starting Position: Sit on the edge of a bench with a dumbbell in each hand. Lie back, keeping the dumbbells close to your chest. Keep your palms facing each other, your hips and lower back firmly grounded on the bench, and your feet flat on the floor. Press the weight up while you breathe out, keeping the weight directly over your chest.

Keep the dumbbells parallel to each other. Next, move the dumbbells above your head while keeping your arms straight until your elbows are directly above your forehead.

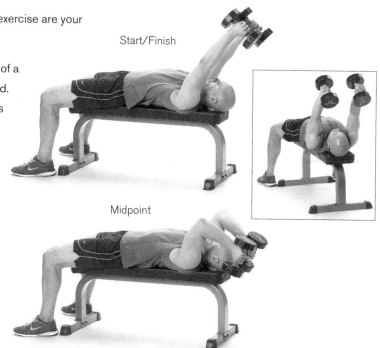

Start/Finish

Midpoint

The Exercise: Slowly lower the dumbbells, bending your arms at your elbows. Stop momentarily when the dumbbells are just above your head. Keeping your elbows stationary, lift the dumbbells up as you straighten your arms. Repeat.

 Tips: Keep your elbows stationary throughout this movement. Do not move your elbows above your face or chest. Keep the dumbbells parallel to each other throughout this movement.

 Focal Point: Draw your attention directly into your triceps, creating the strongest contraction as your arms straighten.

Don't Do: Don't bring the weights directly over your chest between each rep, and do not allow your elbows to shift out to the sides of your shoulders as you lower the dumbbells. Keep your elbows in line with your shoulders.

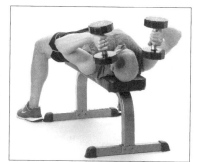

The primary muscles in this exercise are your biceps.

Start/Finish

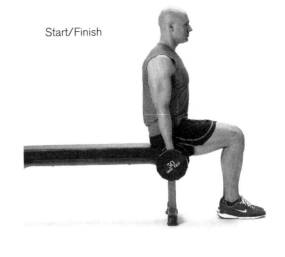

Starting Position: From a seated position, hold two dumbbells, allowing your arms to naturally rest at your sides, palms facing forward (if standing, stand with feet shoulder width apart).

The Exercise: Lift the weights slowly up toward your chest, keeping your elbows directly at your sides from start to finish. Contract the biceps muscle as hard as you can at the top and hold it for a count of one. Then lower the weights for a count of two. One of the best ways to increase the effectiveness of this exercise is to let the weights down slowly. Exhale on the way up and inhale on the way down.

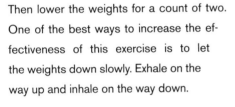

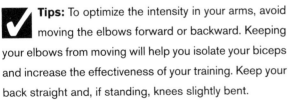

Midpoint

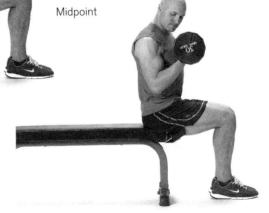

 Tips: To optimize the intensity in your arms, avoid moving the elbows forward or backward. Keeping your elbows from moving will help you isolate your biceps and increase the effectiveness of your training. Keep your back straight and, if standing, knees slightly bent.

Focal Point: Center your attention directly on your biceps. Generate the fullest, tightest contraction at the top of this movement. Maintain a strong contraction of your biceps as you lower the weight.

The primary muscles used in this exercise are your abdominals.

Start/Finish

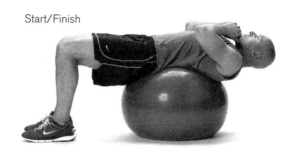

Starting Position: Sit on the ball and slowly walk your feet away until you are comfortably lying back on the ball. With your feet shoulder width apart, put your hands at the sides of your head, underneath your chin, or on your stomach.

Midpoint

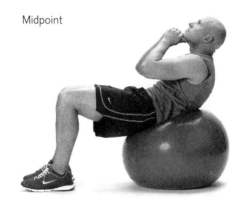

The Exercise: Contract your ab muscles and curl your chest and shoulders up by bringing your sternum toward your pelvis. Keep your chin tucked in to your chest to avoid "jerking" your head up. At the top of this movement, contract your abs as you pause momentarily. Then slowly lower your torso. Repeat.

 Tips: Do not allow your body to fully arch back with the shape of the ball as you begin and end each repetition. This decreases the tension on your abs. Use the ball to support your back and your feet and legs to stabilize the movement.

Focal Point: Focus on the quality of the contraction in the abdominal muscles through slow, controlled movements. Do not be distracted by how much or how little you're moving.

The primary muscle group used in this exercise is your abdominals.

Starting Position: Lie on your back, knees bent and feet together, about six inches above the bench. Put your hands behind your head, gripping on to the sides of the bench.

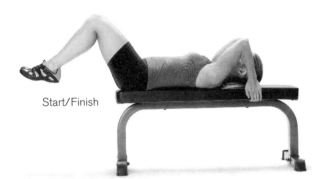

Start/Finish

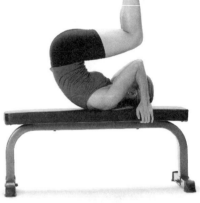

Midpoint

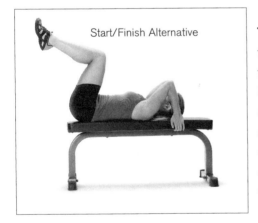

Start/Finish Alternative

The Exercise: Keeping your feet close to your hips, contract your abs while you slowly curl your lower body up toward your shoulders, gradually rolling your hips off the bench. Exhale when you contract the abs on the way up, allowing for a more intense muscle contraction. Keep contracting the abs until your hips and lower back raise off the bench, elevating your hips as high as able. Inhale as you slowly lower your hips back to the starting position. Repeat.

Tips: The slower and more controlled you do this exercise, the better it works. Bring your knees and feet over your core to make this exercise easier; allow your knees and feet to move farther over your hips to increase the difficulty.

Focal Point: Focus on the quality of the contraction in the abdominal muscles through slow, controlled movements. Do not be distracted by how much or how little you're moving.

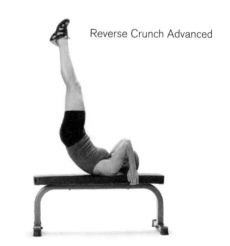

Reverse Crunch Advanced

Reverse Crunch Advanced

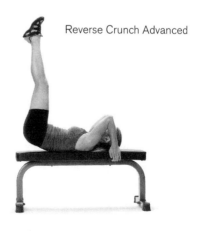

Reverse Crunch Advanced

The primary muscle group used in this exercise is the obliques.

Starting Position: Lie on your back, knees bent, with your feet flat on the floor. Put both hands behind your head.

The Exercise: Contracting your ab muscles, lift your chest and shoulders toward your pelvis. As your upper back rises off the floor, rotate your upper torso toward one side. Pause at the top of this motion, exhaling all of your air before slowly returning to the starting position. Switch sides after you've completed all your reps on one side (do not alternate).

Start/Finish   Midpoint

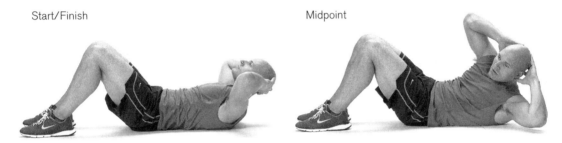

 Tips: In between reps, do not allow your upper back, shoulders, and head to touch the floor. Don't pull on your head or use momentum.

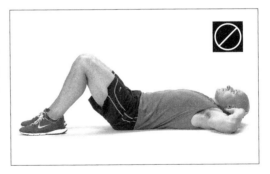

Focal Point: Focus on driving your ribs down toward your hips as you twist.

The primary muscle group used in this exercise is your abdominals.

Starting Position: Lie on your back with your knees bent, feet resting flat on the floor. Gently position your hands behind your head or just below your chin.

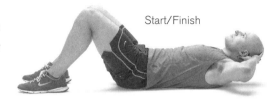
Start/Finish

The Exercise: Contracting your ab muscles and pushing your lower back into the floor, slowly curl your chest and shoulders up by bringing your sternum toward your pelvis, lifting your upper back off the floor. Avoid jerking or pulling your head up and do not sit all the way up. At the top of the movement, contract your abs fully while exhaling all of your air and pressing your lower back into the floor. Pause here for about two seconds. While maintaining the contraction in your abs, slowly lower your chest and shoulders back down, stopping just before your shoulder blades touch the floor. Repeat.

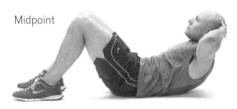
Midpoint

 Tips: Your hands can be used to support your head and neck during this exercise but do not use them for leveraging your body upward. Be sure not to strain your neck, by keeping your chin tucked into your chest throughout the exercise. With focused intensity this "simple" ab exercise can be one of the best ways to transform your midsection. To increase the difficulty of each crunch, you can raise your legs into the air while maintaining a 90-degree bend in your knees.

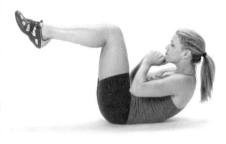

Focal Point: Intensely contract your ab muscles before beginning this movement and throughout this exercise.

Don't Do: Don't allow your shoulder blades, shoulders, and head to completely lower to the ground between each repetition. Avoid moving your head throughout the movement.

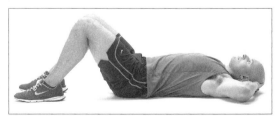

Dumbbell Bench Press

Refer to Monday exercises.

One-Arm Dumbbell Rows

Refer to Thursday exercises.

Dumbbell Side Raises

Refer to Monday exercises.

Lying Dumbbell Triceps Extensions

Refer to Thursday exercises.

Dumbbell Biceps Curls

Refer to Monday exercises.

The primary muscle groups used in this exercise are the quadriceps, hamstrings, hips, and glutes.

Starting Position: Stand with your feet shoulder width apart and your arms resting at your sides.

The Exercise: Step laterally to the right side, opening up your hips, and squat down into your right leg. Keep your left leg straight and your arms out in front of you for balance. Stop when your right leg is parallel with the ground. Pause momentarily before standing up. To return to the starting position, drive forcefully through your right leg. Do not rest at the top of this movement until you've completed your entire set. Do all of your reps on one leg and follow with your other side.

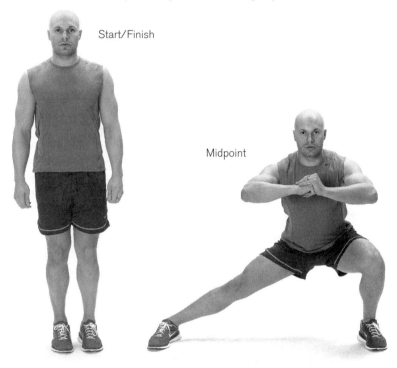

Start/Finish

Midpoint

 Tips: If you are going to use weights, hold one dumbbell in your hand on the same side as you're lunging. As you step into your lunge, pull the dumbbell up and hold it at your hip until returning back to the starting position. Use light dumbbells for this exercise.

Focal Point: Place your focus on driving the heel and ball of your foot forcefully into the ground as if you were jumping off this leg to engage your quad, hamstring, hip, and glute muscles.

An integral part of your FIT Full-Body Saturday workout, and one of the three Cornerstones of Fitness as discussed in Chapter 13, the following stretches provide an introductory stretching program that will increase the flexibility of most of your major muscle groups.

Proper stretching helps increase the length of your muscles and tendons, increases your range of motion, relieves stress, and helps prevent injuries. It is important to take your time entering into and coming out of each stretch. Do not jump up out of the movements. Also, be sure not to bounce during your stretching; instead, slowly deepen each stretch and hold it by taking your time, releasing your breath slowly and steadily as you increase your flexibility.

Each of the following stretches should be held for 30 to 60 seconds. If you are a beginner, start with 30 seconds, working your way toward 60 seconds as your flexibility increases over time.

Toe Touches

With your feet approximately shoulder width apart (or closer), and with knees slightly bent, bend at the waist and reach your hands down the front of your legs. Throughout this stretch, keep your legs straight (not locked) and back flat, in particular your lower back.

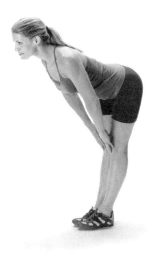
Basic Stretch Start

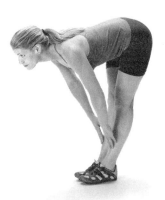
Basic Stretch Finish

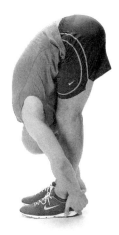
Advanced

While resting on both knees on a padded surface, start by stepping your left leg forward in a lunging movement. Leave your right knee firmly on the ground along with your right toe. Focus on keeping your hips "square," with your shoulders evenly facing forward. Support yourself with both hands on the floor or rest your hands on your left knee as you raise your torso up, increasing the depth of the stretch. Be sure not to allow your knee to move in front of your ankle. Switch sides.

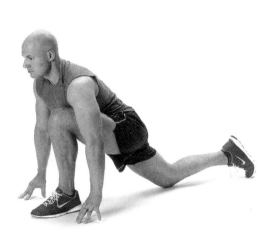
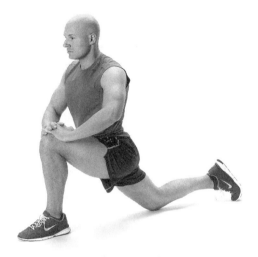

Basic Stretch Start   Basic Stretch Finish

Lie facedown making a 90-degree angle with your right arm, then shift your arm up several inches so your hand is even with the top of your head. Next, roll up toward your right side and right shoulder while keeping your right hand in place, supporting yourself with your left hand. You should feel this gently stretch both your shoulder and your chest. To deepen the stretch, push farther up onto your right side. To lessen the stretch, lower yourself down toward the ground with your left hand. Switch sides.

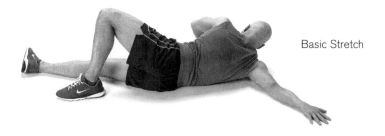

Basic Stretch

Additional Angle

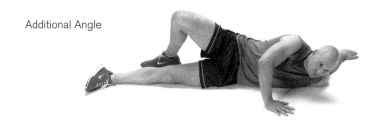

Lie on your back with your arms in a T position out to your sides. Shift your hips to the right approximately three inches. Lift your right knee and right foot up into the air, creating a 90-degree angle at your right hip as well as at your right knee. Next, allow your right leg to roll across your body. As you allow your knee to approach the ground, rotate your hips with your right leg. As you deepen your stretch, keep both hands and shoulders on the ground. Switch sides.

Basic Stretch Start

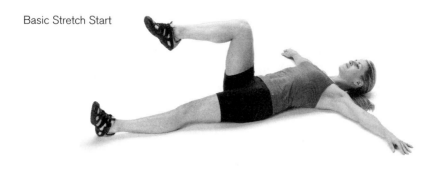

Basic Stretch Finish

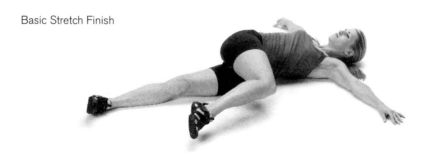

Additional Angle

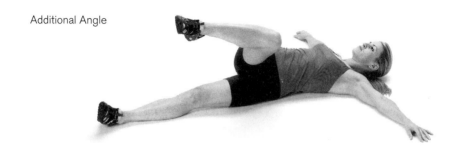

Lie on your stomach. Come up onto your elbows, arching your back and opening the chest, and gently lift your chin. Keep your heels together. To deepen this stretch, bring your hands directly underneath your shoulders and push up until your arms are straight. Focus on arching your upper and middle back in addition to your lower back.

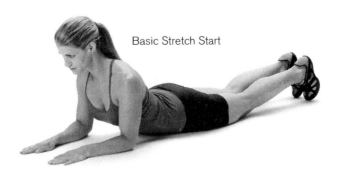

Basic Stretch Start

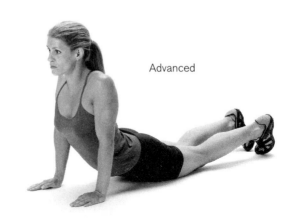

Advanced

Bring your knees and feet together on a padded surface and sit back on your heels. Slowly walk your hands forward, allowing your torso to rest on your thighs. Let your armpits drop toward the ground as you open up your chest and shoulders. To deepen the stretch, continue to walk your arms forward until your hips are directly above your knees. Next, rise up onto your fingertips, again allowing your armpits to drop toward the ground.

Basic Stretch Start

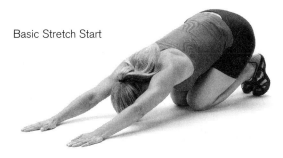

Basic Stretch Finish

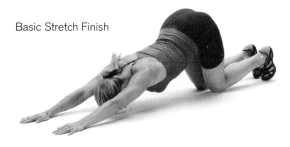

Advanced

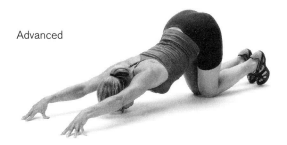

Workout Trackers

Monday **PUSH** Chest | Shoulders | Triceps + Biceps

DATE _____ WK#_____ START TIME _____ FINISH TIME _____

	SET	EXERCISE	TBS	PLANNED WEIGHT/REPS	TiL	ACTUAL WEIGHT/REPS	AiL
CHEST	1	Dumbbell Bench Press		/12	2	/	
	2		60	/10	3	/	
	3		60	/8	4	/	
	4		60	/8+	(5)	/	
	5	Dumbbell Flyes	60	/10	4	/	
	6		0	/10+	(5)	/	
SHOULDERS	7	Dumbbell Side Raises	60	/12	2	/	
	8		60	/10	3	/	
	9		60	/10	4	/	
	10		0	/8+	(5)	/	
ARMS	11	Dumbbell Triceps Kickbacks	60	/12	2	/	
	12		60	/10	3	/	
	13		60	/8	4	/	
	14		0	/8+	(5)	/	
	15	Dumbbell Biceps Curls	60	/12	2	/	
	16		60	/10	3	/	
	17		60	/8	4	/	
	18		0	/8+	(5)	/	

POST-WORKOUT   **1** RECORD   **2** PROJECT   **3** REFLECT

★ = DROP-SET   + = TO FAILURE SET |TBS| = TIME *BEFORE* SET (Secs) |TiL| = TARGET INTENSITY LEVEL |AiL| = ACTUAL INTENSITY LEVEL

HIIT/ABS

Tuesday   HIIT | ABS

DATE _____ WK#_____ START TIME _____ FINISH TIME_____

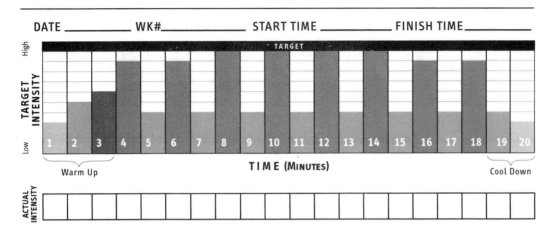

SET	EXERCISE	PLANNED REPS	ACTUAL REPS
1	Swiss Ball Ab Crunches (30 Seconds Rest Between Sets)	12–15	
2		12–15	
3		12–15	
4	Reverse Crunches (30 Seconds Rest Between Sets)	12–15	
5		12–15	
6		12–15	
7	Cross Crunches (30 Seconds Rest Between Sets)	12–15	
8		12–15	
9		12–15	

(ABS)

POST-WORKOUT   ① RECORD   ② PROJECT   ③ REFLECT

STRENGTH FOR LIFE WORKOUT TRACKER

Wednesday　　　　　　**LEGS**　　　Quads | Hamstrings | Calves

DATE _____ WK#_____ START TIME _____ FINISH TIME _____

	SET	EXERCISE	TBS	PLANNED WEIGHT/REPS	TiL	ACTUAL WEIGHT/REPS	AiL
LEGS/QUADS	1	Dumbbell Step Lunges		/12	2	/	
	2		60	/10	3	/	
	3		60	/8	4	/	
	4		60	/8+	(5)	/	
	5	Dumbbell Squats	60	/10	4	/	
	6		0	/10+	(5)	/	
HAMSTRINGS	7	Dumbbell Straight-Leg Deadlifts	60	/12	2	/	
	8		60	/10	3	/	
	9		60	/8	4	/	
	10		0	/8+	(5)	/	
	11	Dumbbell Sumo Squats	60	/12	4	/	
	12		0	/12+	(5)	/	
CALVES	13	Dumbbell Single-Leg Calf Raises	60	/12	2	/	
	14		0	/12	3	/	
	15		0	/12	4	/	
	16		0	/12+	(5)	/	

POST-WORKOUT　　①RECORD　　②PROJECT　　③REFLECT

★ = DROP-SET   + = TO FAILURE SET |TBS| = TIME *BEFORE* SET (Secs) |TiL| = TARGET INTENSITY LEVEL |AiL| = ACTUAL INTENSITY LEVEL

Thursday   **PULL**   Back | Rear Delts | Triceps + Biceps

DATE _____ WK# _____ START TIME _____ FINISH TIME _____

	SET	EXERCISE	TBS	PLANNED WEIGHT/REPS	TiL	ACTUAL WEIGHT/REPS	AiL
BACK	1	One-Arm Dumbbell Rows		/12	2	/	
	2		60	/10	3	/	
	3		60	/8	4	/	
	4		60	/8+	⑤	/	
	5	Dumbbell Pullovers	60	/10	4	/	
	6		0	/10+	⑤	/	
SHOULDERS	7	Reverse Dumbbell Flyes	60	/12	2	/	
	8		60	/10	3	/	
	9		60	/10	4	/	
	10		0	/8+	⑤	/	
ARMS	11	Lying Dumbbell Triceps Extensions	60	/12	2	/	
	12		60	/10	3	/	
	13		60	/8	4	/	
	14		0	/8+	⑤	/	
	15	Dumbbell Biceps Curls	60	/12	2	/	
	16		60	/10	3	/	
	17		60	/8	4	/	
	18		0	/8+	⑤	/	

POST-WORKOUT   ❶ RECORD   ❷ PROJECT   ❸ REFLECT

★ = DROP-SET   + = TO FAILURE SET |TBS| = TIME *BEFORE* SET (Secs) |TiL| = TARGET INTENSITY LEVEL |AiL| = ACTUAL INTENSITY LEVEL

HIIT/ABS

Friday

HIIT | ABS

DATE _____ WK#_____ START TIME _____ FINISH TIME _____

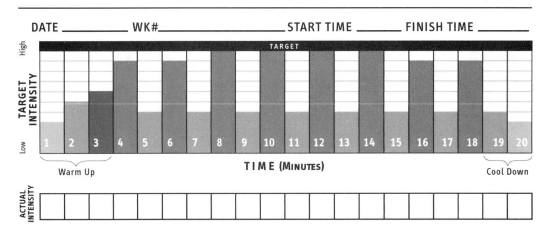

TARGET INTENSITY

High

Low

TARGET

1 2 3 4 5 6 7 8 9 10 11 12 13 14 15 16 17 18 19 20

Warm Up

TIME (MINUTES)

Cool Down

ACTUAL INTENSITY

SET	EXERCISE	PLANNED REPS	ACTUAL REPS
1	Ab Crunches (30 Seconds Rest Between Sets)	12–15	
2		12–15	
3		12–15	
4	Reverse Crunches (30 Seconds Rest Between Sets)	12–15	
5		12–15	
6		12–15	
7	Cross Crunches (30 Seconds Rest Between Sets)	12–15	
8		12–15	
9		12–15	

ABS

POST-WORKOUT   ① RECORD   ② PROJECT   ③ REFLECT

Saturday

FIT CIRCUIT

Total Body

DATE _____ WK#_____ START TIME _____ FINISH TIME _____

	EXERCISE	TiL	CIRCUIT 1 WEIGHT/REP	AiL	CIRCUIT 2 WEIGHT/REP	AiL	CIRCUIT 3 WEIGHT/REP	AiL
1	Dumbbell Bench Press	3	/		/		/	
2	One-Arm Dumbbell Row	3	/		/		/	
3	Dumbbell Side Raises	3	/		/		/	
4	Lying Dumbbell Triceps Extensions	4	/		/		/	
5	Biceps Curls	4	/		/		/	
6	Sidestep Lunges	4	/		/		/	

OPTIONAL

No rest between each exercise. 2–3 minute recovery between circuits. 3rd set is optional.

	EXERCISE	TARGET DURATION	ACTUAL DURATION
1	Toe Touches	30–60 Seconds	
2	Lunge (each side)	30–60 Seconds	
3	Flye Stretch (each side)	30–60 Seconds	
4	Twists (each side)	30–60 Seconds	
5	Seal Stretch	30–60 Seconds	
6	Cat Stretch	30–60 Seconds	

FIT STRETCH

POST-WORKOUT ❶ RECORD ❷ PROJECT ❸ REFLECT

|TiL| = TARGET INTENSITY LEVEL |AiL| = ACTUAL INTENSITY LEVEL

Gym Alternatives

STRENGTH EXCHANGE

In support of your Transformation, the Strength for Life program is designed to leverage the many benefits offered by dumbbells (see Chapter 11). Dumbbells are especially advantageous for those who train at home and make for an efficient workout.

	DUMBBELL EXERCISE		GYM EQUIPMENT ALTERNATIVE	
CHEST	Dumbbell Press		Barbell Bench Press	
	Dumbbell Flyes		Cable Flyes	
SHOULDERS	Dumbbell Side Raises		Cable Side Raises	
TRICEPS	Dumbbell Triceps Kickbacks		Triceps Cable Push-Downs	
	Lying Dumbbell Extensions		Dips	
BICEPS	Dumbbell Biceps Curls		Barbell Biceps Curls	
	Concentration Curls		Cable Biceps Curls	

STRENGTH EXCHANGE

For those with access to a well-stocked gym or fitness center, and seek variety, this chart offers you some simple, direct substitutions. Make the exchanges that work best for you. Enjoy the strength!

DUMBBELL EXERCISE	GYM EQUIPMENT ALTERNATIVE	
One-Arm Dumbbell Row	Cable Long Rows	BACK
Dumbbell Pullovers	Lat Cable Pulldowns	
Dumbbell Squats	Leg Press	
Dumbbell Lunges	Leg Extensions	LEGS
Dumbbell Straight-Leg Deadlifts	Leg Curls	
Dumbbell Single-Leg Calf Raises	Calf Machine	
Crunch	Cable Crunch	ABS

Glossary

Aerobic. This term means "with oxygen." Exercise where oxygen is used primarily to generate energy in the muscles. This includes activities like jogging, biking, stair climbers, or any exercise performed at moderate levels of intensity for extended periods of time.

Aging. There are two types of aging: *chronological,* measured in calendar years, and *biological,* measured through various markers of biological changes. What this means is that the age on your driver's license is simply a rough estimate of your biological age. Genetic and lifestyle factors influence people to age at different rates, biologically.

Amino Acid. The nutrient building blocks from which proteins are made. Muscle tissue, hormones, neurotransmitters in your brain, your immune system antibodies, and the many enzymes in your body are all made from amino acids.

Anabolic. The metabolic process by which cells repair and grow; for example, building lean muscle. It often refers to an overall positive body state prime for "building."

Anaerobic. Exercise where energy is created in the muscle primarily without oxygen. This occurs when there are short bursts of power, when intensity is high and the duration is short, generally less than one minute, such as in strength training.

Base Camp. An integrated 12-day conditioning phase in *Strength for Life* that is essential to fully prepare your body and mind for maximum results from the strenuous and challenging 12-week Transformation Training Camp. In the absence of this vital preparation, a significant percentage of people have failed to complete a 12-week Transformation.

Breakfast. The first and most important meal of your day. It *breaks* the night's *fast*.

Breathing. The act of drawing air into and expelling it from the lungs in order to capture essential oxygen. Breathing is the only bodily process that is both passive (automatic) and active (under your control). It is a point of contact between the external and the internal and can serve as an anchor for focus and stability during your training.

Calories. The amount of usable energy a food contains. Protein and carbohydrates are known to contain four calories per gram, while fats contain nine calories per gram. Calorie consumption has a significant impact on metabolism and whether you add or subtract fat or muscle.

Carbohydrates (Carbs). The macronutrient primarily responsible for storage and transport of energy. An essential component of every meal, as carbohydrates also help transport proteins to your vital organs.

Cardio. Exercises and the related equipment intended for cardiovascular fitness and endurance training.

Catabolic. The metabolic process of breaking down muscle tissue for energy. Poor nutrition (eating), stress, and lack of sleep often combine to produce a chronic state where the body is breaking down. This condition can lead to low energy and excess fat storage and numerous other serious imbalances in hormones. Many people attempt to self-medicate this condition by consuming more caffeine and sugars.

Concentric. The lifting phase of an exercise when a muscle contracts and the weight is lifted up against the force of gravity.

Consumption to Freedom. The higher relationship with food characterized by an increasing awareness of how food impacts your body and mind *after* consumption. This relation to food enhances your freedom to choose foods that are good for you, elevating productivity and providing high and lasting energy.

Cornerstones of Fitness. A *Strength for Life* system for sustaining and energizing a lifetime of fitness. This system is personal and dynamic, integrating the fitness components of Strength, Stamina, and Stretching (Flexibility) into seasons of training for an annual peak that can keep you at your best for life.

Cravings to Consumption. The most common relationship with food characterized by using food in reaction to cravings that are the result of physiological or emotional desires, not by physiological needs.

Diet. A test of willpower in which one attempts to regulate and control food intake, usually in order to lose weight. The experience is often one of deprivation and suffering, leading to revolt. Dieting is counterintuitive as it is focused on "being less" rather than enhancing life.

Discipline. The effort intended to produce a specific pattern of behavior.

Drop Set. The second set of two sets of an exercise done in a consecutive manner with no rest between the first and second. The drop set is performed using less weight than used in the first set.

Dumbbell. A free weight used in strength training that is designed to be held in one hand.

Eccentric. The lowering phase of an exercise when the muscle is lengthened and the weight is lowered.

Energy. The strength and vitality required to sustain physical and mental activity. Energy is found in the nutrients from balanced, nourishing meals and is enhanced through your training.

Essential Fats. The good fat—a source of essential fatty acids required for healthy skin, hair, and cell functioning, organ insulation, temperature regulation, and energy storage. The omega-3s, omega-6s, and omega-9s that help you stay healthy, enjoy ample energy, and lose fat.

Exercise. An activity usually requiring nominal physical effort and carried out in the hopes of sustaining or improving health and fitness. Exercise often lacks goals and intensity and thus is less productive and transformative than *training,* which is focused.

Focus Intensity Index. A five-level scale for rating and targeting your training intensity in *Strength for Life,* with 1 being the lowest level intensity and 5 being Peak Intensity.

Focus Intensity Training (FIT). An integrated form of strength training pioneered by Shawn Phillips and featured in *Strength for Life* that combines physical and mental strength techniques in training that can enhance enjoyment and results. FIT embraces the Eastern philosophies found in yoga and martial arts traditions with a Western practice of strength training.

Food. The stuff you eat that contains protein, carbohydrates, fats, and other nutrients. Food is *not* just anything you can put into your mouth and eat. The ultimate purpose of food is for nourishment for your body and mind.

Freedom. The clarity and strength to choose what best serves your life and the greatest good for all.

Full Strength. The world's finest, most premium total-nutrition shake designed not simply to deliver protein, but as a complete, performance-balanced meal. Its Performance Balance technology provides sustained levels of high energy for body and mind. In a scientific study at a prestigious university, Full Strength was shown to significantly enhance fat loss, promote muscle gain, and improve numerous indicators of vitality and wellness in just ten weeks. To learn more, visit: www.FullStrength.com.

Goal. A specific, measurable, and desired outcome that has a clearly defined time frame for achievement.

Habit. Instinctive behavioral patterns and natural tendencies.

Health. The state of being free from illness or injury.

High Intensity Interval Training (HIIT). A highly effective form of cardio training specifically designed to maximize fat loss and minimize time without cannibalizing lean muscle.

Intention. The specific purpose, end, or aim to accomplish. One's thoughtfulness or deliberate goal directedness.

Lean Muscle. A more glamorous and alluring way to say "muscle." Muscle is not just for appearance, but a vital part of a strong and healthy body.

Macronutrients. The nutrients that together provide the majority of metabolic energy. The three macronutrients are carbohydrates, proteins, and fats.

Meal. A balanced and properly portioned grouping of food at a specific time. Macro- and micronutrients are balanced in response to the demands placed on the body.

Metabolism. The process by which your body combines nutrients with oxygen to produce the energy required to keep you alive.

Micronutrients. The vitamins, minerals, and other essential elements that support and/or enhance life. These are delivered in small quantities and derived from food.

Momentary Muscular Fatigue. The point at which you can no longer complete another repetition with proper form.

Motivation. The reason(s) one has for acting or taking action; the general drive, desire, or willingness to do something. There are at least four stages of motivation: obligation, desire, enjoyment, and Mastery.

Neurotransmitter. The master control switches in your brain that relay, amplify, and modulate signals between a neuron and another cell. These include dopamine, serotonin, and norepinephrine, which control drive, mood, and excitement. An imbalance of neurotransmitters can result in low energy and lead to cravings for foods that are ultimately detrimental to your wellness and life.

Nutrition. The nourishment necessary for health, strength, and growth.

Nutrition Shake. An engineered source of nutrition that combines a blend of protein, carbohydrates, fats, vitamins, minerals, water, for the purpose of increasing nutrient intake. Nutrition shakes are best supplied in powder, where you add water. They come in various grades, and are not all made with premium quality ingredients.

Nutritional Awareness. The master nutritional strategy, a knowledge of both how food leaves you feeling after consumption and why you have chosen to consume a certain food in the first place.

Nutritional Freedom. The freedom to eat what's good for you because you choose to, not because you're on a diet. It is acquired through the process of strengthening Nutritional Awareness.

Protein. This essential macronutrient of primary importance is composed of amino acids, provides structural or mechanical functions for cells, and plays a role in cellular communication and immune system functioning. It's also been shown to enhance metabolism and provide greater lasting satiety than carbohydrates or fats, which means you stay free from hunger longer.

Rep. Short for "repetition." The movement of the weight through an exercise's full range of motion from start to midpoint to finish. A repetition includes both the lifting and lowering of the weight.

Ritual. A conscious, positive, life-enhancing behavioral pattern intended to improve one's functioning.

S Curve. An elevation in life, strength, and energy of body and mind through integrated training. The emphasis is to move from a sustaining life of *health* to an abundant life of *strength*.

Set. The number of repetitions (reps) of an exercise considered to comprise one set (e.g., 12 reps is one set).

Shake Break. A brief five-minute break for refueling your body and recharging your mind that is integrated in the Full Strength premium nutrition program. Designed by Shawn Phillips to be a part of the Full Strength protocol. See www.ShakeBreak.com for more information.

Stamina. The enduring physical or mental energy and strength that allows people to do something for a long time.

Strength. The abundant energy and capacity to be a force for change in your world. It's more than health; it's the abundance of energy, power, and confidence.

Strength Training. A positive life-enhancing form of focus, results-producing exercise that strengthens, shapes, and defines the body and energizes the mind. It is most often associated with weight training but is also found in various forms of yoga and simple body weight movements.

Stretch. The activity of gradually applying tensile force to lengthen muscles to increase the flexibility and range of motion within a joint, help prevent injury, and increase blood circulation.

Touch Training. A specific technique of FIT that generates stronger, more focused contractions in the muscles being trained.

Training. A focused, purposeful, goal-directed mind-set brought to each exercise and characterized by an intense drive to achieve.

Transformation. Significant *and* lasting change in your body and mind. A "Transformation" is a 12-week period of intense training designed to facilitate strength gains, physique changes, and improved cardio-vascular functioning.

Transformation Training Camp (TTC). The signature *Strength for Life* Transformation 12-week program.

Turning Point. An opportunity for change, accepted. Whether you accept the opportunity for change determines whether you're at or "in" a turning point.

Vision. An optimistic view of where you want to be in the future. A "true north" or ideal toward which you aspire.

Weight Lifting. A type of training for sculpting and shaping the body while developing the strength, power, endurance, and/or size of muscles, using the force of gravity in the form of weighted bars, dumbbells, or weight stacks.

Willpower. The strength of the faculty by which a person decides on and initiates action.

Wogging. An extremely low-intensity walk that occasionally mixes in a slight jog.

Workout. The performance of a physical activity for a set period of time, or predetermined goal, or for the purpose of enhancing fitness, health, and strength.

Acknowledgments

The collection of words, thoughts, concepts, and images that create the sentences, paragraphs, and charts that comprise this book reflect a life's work and an extraordinary commitment to creating the best book for you.

While I will be forever credited as the author of *Strength for Life,* this book is by no means a solo effort. This book owes its existence to a team of people. And I wish to express my sincere appreciation to all those who have contributed to bringing the book to life and to all those, mentioned or not, who have contributed to my life experience and the wealth of knowledge shared in this book.

First and foremost I thank my family: my wife Angie, who has been both a vital contributor to this book with her meticulous eye for editing and a patient supporter during the marathon months of writing, late nights, and long days. And to my son Nathaniel, who kept me sane, not buying into the seriousness of all this and preferring to pull me into a game or some Hot Wheels or to just "bonk" me.

As contributions go, none have been greater or more appreciated than my brother Bill, who has played numerous roles throughout our forty-some years together: a training partner, business associate, supporter, confidant, and, most important, my friend. His pioneering work, which has changed millions of lives, made this book a possibility. Thank you for sharing *your* strength so courageously for all these years.

Throughout my years of writing and life, my mom, Suzanne, has been a steady source of support, encouragement, and humor. My sister, Shelly, who's always able to find the bright spot and locate the way forward: Perhaps no one has been a better source of stability throughout the years than her. And no recognition of contribution or family would be complete without a big thanks to my dad, BP, whose spirit, tenacity, drive, and wisdom is with me each and every day. Your presence is deeply missed by your children.

I want to thank the superhero of literary agents, David Black, for encouraging me to create this book and for masterfully orchestrating its growth from concept to reality. Also, my editor at Ballantine Books, Caroline Sutton, and the entire team at Random House and Ballantine for their enthusiasm, commitment, encouragement, and ultimately for their patience as I performed my own reenactment of the painting of the Sistine Chapel.

To the many people who reviewed chapters in development, I wish to express my thanks. A few whose contribution stands out include my friends and confidants who have graced my life over the last few years in my EO Forum; many thanks to Bill, Danny, David, Doug, Jason, Patrick, Peter, Matt, Tyler, and Scott for their support, encouragement, friendship, and for always inspiring and challenging me. For lending their full attention to the many renditions throughout this process, I thank: Monty Miranda, Blake Frye, John Basso, Tom Terwilliger, Ken Jacobs, and Brian Johnson. And in the memory of my friend and role model for living at full strength, Bobby Blanchard.

To my friend and collaborator Brett Thomas, thank you for your invaluable contribution to illuminating Focus Intensity Training. And to Stagen Institute for the clarity, support, and guidance along the path. To my friend Eric Hillman, thank you for all that you've been in my life for the last decade. Many thanks to Dennis Lane for lending his buoyant energy, skilled eye, and lens for the crystal-clear photography. To my friend and fellow champion for strength and fitness, Jon Benson, thank you. Many thanks to Melissa Edwards for polishing the visuals that are so critical to the communication, Chris Monck for his assistance on layout, and Dawn Terwilliger for her outstanding modeling and direction in the exercise photos.

I wish to extend extra-special recognition and deep appreciation to my friend and associate Tom Bilella ("Doctor Tom") for stunning clarity and real world wisdom, what can only be garnered from years on the front lines, changing lives. I value your knowledge, energy, and passion, but most of all I am proud to call you my friend. I look forward to changing the world together.

My most profound gratitude to Ken Wilber for the inspiration and guidance I have found throughout the years in his work; he has elevated and energized me in his presence. And to the Integral Institute, which has embraced me along with my FIT practice, providing fertile ground for its evolution in the real world. To all those I've guided and been guided by in the retreats, it's been a pleasure and honor. And to the entire team at *What Is Enlightenment?* magazine, who have helped spread the word about FIT; the new path to strength.

And finally but most important, I extend gratitude beyond the perceived bounds of this universe to my "Full Strength" team at Phillips Performance Nutrition, including Jodi Kostelnik, who nearly single-handedly kept the Full Strength flowing for the final four months of this project while the rest of us pushed each day for the finish line. And to Mike Metz for his hands, which are faster than the eye. To the dynamic duo of Tom Bottagaro and Rob McNamara, I can find no words to adequately express my heartfelt appreciation for the way you both committed to this project and carried it on your shoulders. I can only imagine that like any soldiers who have fought shoulder to shoulder, you have both earned my deepest respect. I have no doubt that we have all come through this challenge stronger.

Index

ABOUT THE AUTHOR

A Colorado native, SHAWN PHILLIPS is an author, entrepreneur, and world respected expert in the area of strength and fitness. For the past two decades he has helped hundreds of thousands of people including business leaders, professional athletes, and numerous celebrities, look great, feel great, and enjoy life at full strength.

After helping to build some of the leading names in performance nutrition, including EAS, Shawn created the premium nutrition shake *Full Strength*®, clinically proven to enhance fat loss, build lean muscle, and improve numerous markers of optimum health. Shawn has focused his considerable passion on transforming the strength and fitness of our country.

An ambassador for transformation and personal freedom, Shawn is the creator of *Focus Intensity Training*™, a system that integrates body and mind, blending the depth of eastern traditions with the western form and function of strength training. He founded the Coalition for Strength, a nonprofit organization to share the benefits of living with strength and inspire people of all ages. He has also served as faculty and member of the Integral Institute, a leader in the field of human potential.

While known by many for his signature "six-pack abs," and his brilliant clarity and inspiring vision, Shawn is better known by his family, close friends, and associates as a focused hardworking man with a kind heart and an intense passion for helping people live extraordinary lives. Shawn currently lives in the foothills of Colorado with his wife Angie, their son, Nathaniel, and daughter, Lilly.

ABOUT THE TYPE

This book was set in Fairfield, the first typeface from the hand of the distinguished American artist and engraver Rudolph Ruzicka (1883–1978). Ruzicka was born in Bohemia and came to America in 1894. He set up his own shop, devoted to wood engraving and printing, in New York in 1913 after a varied career working as a wood engraver, in photoengraving and banknote printing plants, and as an art director and freelance artist. He designed and illustrated many books, and was the creator of a considerable list of individual prints—wood engravings, line engravings on copper, and aquatints.